Changing U.S. Health Care

**The Eisenhower Center for the
Conservation of Human Resources
• Studies in Health Policy •**

Changing U.S. Health Care

A Study of Four Metropolitan Areas

Eli Ginzberg,
Howard S. Berliner,
and Miriam Ostow

*with E. Richard Brown, Hardy D. Loe, Jr.,
and J. Warren Salmon*

WESTVIEW PRESS
BOULDER • SAN FRANCISCO • OXFORD

The Eisenhower Center for the Conservation of Human Resources Studies in Health Policy

Copyright © 1993 by The Eisenhower Center for the Conservation of Human Resources, Columbia University

Published in 1993 in the United States of America by Westview Press, Inc., 5500 Central Avenue, Boulder, Colorado 80301-2877, and in the United Kingdom by Westview Press, 36 Lonsdale Road, Summertown, Oxford OX2 7EW

Library of Congress Cataloging-in-Publication Data
Changing U.S. health care : a study of four metropolitan areas / Eli
    Ginzberg, Howard S. Berliner, Miriam Ostow, and associates ... [et al.].
        p.   cm.— (Conservation of human resources studies in health policy)
    Municipal Health Services Program (U.S.)
    ISBN 0-8133-8544-X
    1. Urban health—United States—Case studies.   2. Medical care—
New York (N.Y.)   3. Medical care—Illinois— Chicago.   4. Medical
care—California—Los Angeles.   5. Medical care—Texas—Houston.
I. Ginzberg, Eli, 1911–   .   II. Berliner, Howard S., 1949–
III. Ostow, Miriam, 1920–   .   IV. Series.
    [DNLM: 1. Municipal Health Services Program (U.S.)   2. Delivery of
Health Care—Chicago.   3. Delivery of Health Care—Los Angeles.
4. Delivery of Health Care—New York.   5. Delivery of Health Care—
Texas.   WA 546 AA1 C4]
RA566.3.C48   1993
362.1' 0973—dc20
DNLM/DLC
for Library of Congress   91-47575
                                                                                                          CIP

Printed and bound in the United States of America

(∞)   The paper used in this publication meets the requirements
        of the American National Standard for Permanence of Paper
        for Printed Library Materials Z39.48-1984.

10   9   8   7   6   5   4   3   2   1

Contents

Tables

Acknowledgments

In the preparation of this volume, which is an assessment of the changes that transpired during the decade of the 1980s in the health care systems of New York City, Chicago, Houston, and Los Angeles—and by inference those of other metropolitan areas in the United States—The Eisenhower Center for the Conservation of Human Resources, Columbia University, has incurred a debt of gratitude to numerous organizations and individuals.

We wish first to acknowledge the confidence and the generosity of The Robert Wood Johnson Foundation in providing support for a three-year research program that promised no clearly defined outcome, only the gathering and analysis of current data, using traditional and non-traditional techniques, to ascertain how the urban American was faring in terms of health and health care needs and how well the local governments, hospitals, health departments, physicians, and others were discharging their responsibilities as providers and financers of care at the end of a decade of change, uncertainty and mounting anxiety. Our success in identifying new and emerging trends and distinguishing priorities and effective interventions is the measure of the usefulness of the research for policy guidance.

The soundness and the incisiveness of the assessments and the validity of the conclusions are largely attributable to our field colleagues and co-authors, who conducted the research in their individual cities, cooperated with our rigorous reporting schedules, critically reviewed the findings and interpretations, and refined the manuscript that we jointly produced. Less apparent are the assistance of the staffs of our field colleagues and the contributions of the many agencies, public officials, administrators, bureaucrats, health care professionals, allied health professionals, policy analysts, legislators, corporate personnel, employers, journalists, and countless others whose inputs of information and opinion, documented and oral, are the substrate of the book. Some have been identified, others not, but they all know who they are and we thank them.

Finally, the preparation of the manuscript for publication is the work of the support staff of The Eisenhower Center for the Conservation of Human Resources: Shoshana Vasheetz, Brian Canivan, Gregory Grove, and

Sylvia Leef, whose technical skills, meticulous attention to detail, patience and good humor have seen this work from first draft through countless revisions to its final form. They were joined by Cynthia Saunders, graduate research assistant, who performed the laborious task of reviewing the edited text for accuracy and form and saw the manuscript through the exacting process of publication.

Eli Ginzberg
Howard S. Berliner
Miriam Ostow

1

Health Care in the 1980s: Overview and Focus

Eli Ginzberg

The decade of the 1980s promised basic reform in the provision of health care services. Ronald Reagan, newly elected to the presidency on a pledge to minimize the role of government in domestic affairs, committed his administration to the pursuit of free market strategies as the panacea for the costliness and inefficiency besetting the nation's health care system. Official and private rhetoric was replete with proposals for systemic change fueled by the competitive forces that would be unleashed by deregulation. Some of the more radical predictions that gained currency were the demise of fee-for-service medicine with the growth of health maintenance organizations (HMOs); the domination of the hospital sector by for-profit hospital chains; and the expansion of hospital systems and networks to a point where virtually all health care in the United States would be controlled by just ten mega-chains.

As is explicit in its title, this book assesses the changes that actually occurred in the U.S. system of health care during the 1980s through the mirror of the nation's four largest metropolitan centers: New York, Chicago, Houston, and Los Angeles. The authors contrast the rhetoric and predictions of the period with the reality faced by the health care system.

This introductory chapter presents an overview of major transformations in the delivery of health care during the 1980s. It provides the contextual background for the detailed analysis of the experiences of the four metropolitan areas (henceforth designated by the colloquial "metros") that is the subject of the book.

The 1980s began with the nation suffering from severe inflation, a worsening federal budget deficit, and a health care system increasingly out of control. President Jimmy Carter's efforts to regulate hospital expenditures had been rejected by Congress in favor of the American Hospital Associa-

1

tion's Voluntary Effort (VE) program, which enjoyed some initial success in moderating rising total hospital outlays but then faltered.

The new administration of Ronald Reagan convinced Congress to retrench on federal outlays for Medicaid and a variety of grant-in-aid programs for health. In 1981 the administration and Congress agreed to reduce Medicaid payments during each of the succeeding three years. As partial compensation for the reduction in federal funding, the states were granted considerably broader scope in the administration of the Medicaid program and were given greater discretion over the use of the grant-in-aid monies.

The initial response to cutbacks in federal funding for Medicaid, accompanied by the transfer to the states of broadened responsibility for program administration, produced one definitive change during the 1980s—namely, considerably reduced health care coverage for the poor and the near poor. In the mid-1970s, approximately two out of every three persons with incomes at or below the federal poverty level were enrolled in Medicaid. By the mid-1980s the proportion declined to two out of five. Most states had responded to the 1981 federal cuts by thinning the number of enrollees and by restricting the range of services that they provided.

To complete the Medicaid story: Alarmed by the unfavorable record of the United States in infant mortality, Congress resorted in 1984 to mandating expanded Medicaid coverage for low-income pregnant women and children. Initially, the states acquiesced more or less agreeably with these actions, but toward the end of the decade the steep increases in their Medicaid outlays and their deteriorating budgetary positions led the governors to petition Congress not once but twice to refrain from further mandates. Although at decade's end the proportion of the poor enrolled in Medicaid was closer to one in two, the ratio was still well below what it had been fifteen years earlier. It is noteworthy that this serious decrease in the proportion of the poor covered by Medicaid occurred with little public attention and even less state and local response; virtually the only response was Congress' concern with improved services for pregnant women and young children. The poor had few spokespersons and fewer allies able and willing to agitate on their behalf.

If one turns from the poor to the well-insured population—those groups that enjoyed good health benefits by virtue of either employment or Medicare coverage—it appears that the decade ended much as it had begun: about two out of every three Americans had broad and deep coverage and had to pay very little—less than 25 percent of their health care costs—out-of-pocket, primarily for dental services, drugs, and nursing home care.

But the foregoing may present too optimistic a picture. It fails to take note of the growing numbers of persons with neither public nor private insurance, estimated to have reached up to 35 million by the end of the decade, and of another 15 million or more with shallow insurance coverage. As the 1980s drew to a close, a large number of individuals found themselves locked into their jobs for fear that they would be unable because of prior or existing medical conditions to obtain coverage in new employment settings.

There was mounting evidence from survey research data that the public was becoming increasingly restive about the U.S. health care system as they learned more about the Canadian and the German systems, which apparently were able to offer more inclusive coverage with lower out-of-pocket payments by beneficiaries. Moreover, a substantial number of American workers found themselves engaged in strikes of shorter or longer duration to prevent their employers from reducing health care benefits or imposing substantial copayments to cover steeply rising premium costs.

Between 1980 and 1989, total health care expenditures increased from $375 to $604 billion (in 1989 constant dollars), or by 61 percent. Hospital admissions, which had climbed steadily until 1982 due to the passage of Medicare and Medicaid, headed downward during the rest of the decade, falling roughly 15 percent below their peak. In the face of such a substantial decline in inpatient admissions, it is striking to find that hospital expenditures rose from $154 billion to $233 billion, or 51 percent. Three explanations are conventionally offered for the paradoxical, steep rise: the increasing sophistication of medical technology and the skilled personnel required for its operation; the increasing number of severely ill patients admitted and treated; and the compensatory increase in the volume of ambulatory care that hospitals provided.

The trend in expenditures for physicians was even more dramatic: Professional earnings rose from $63 billion to $118 billion, or 87 percent. Much of this increase must be attributed to the expanding number of practicing physicians per 100,000 population, which rose from 185 to 240, or by 30 percent. Although the average number of physician-patient contacts per week declined over the decade by approximately 5 percent (having rebounded from a nadir of an 8 percent decrease in 1985), most physicians were able to maintain, even improve, their earnings by raising their fees and providing more intensive services to their patients.

These sharply increased revenues of hospitals and physicians accounted, respectively, for 39 percent and 19 percent—or together just under three out of every five dollars—of total health care outlays in 1989, confronting the principal payers—the federal government, state governments, and employers—with major challenges as they sought to moderate their health care expenditures.

In 1983, the federal government made the first of two major structural changes in the decade by shifting from a cost-based system of hospital reimbursement to a prospective payment system (PPS) in a desperate attempt to brake the runaway costs of inpatient care for Medicare beneficiaries. Analyses of early utilization and cost data indicated that as a result of PPS, outlays for Medicare in 1990 would be $18 billion lower than the amount projected for that year under the prior cost-based reimbursement system.

Paradoxically, in legislating per-case payment by diagnosis related groups (DRGs) the administration and Congress ignored the Reagan administration's ideological commitment to a competitive marketplace solution and relied instead on a rigid system of price controls, which it put into place in late 1983 and has been fine-tuning ever since. Considering the limited experimentation that preceded the legislation, the DRG system has worked with remarkable success. The fact that the original schedule of prospective rates was miscalculated in favor of the hospitals facilitated the adoption of the new system. However, the body charged with overseeing the system—the Prospective Payment Assessment Commission (PROPAC) —has in the intervening years lowered the annual adjustment rate to recapture the earlier overpayments. By the end of the decade, it was generally conceded that Medicare was no longer covering its full share of the costs of hospital care.

In the 1980s, the federal government became increasingly aware of the rapidly rising outlays for physician payments under Medicare B and introduced price freezes and other adjustments aimed at their deceleration. With the passage of fee and volume controls in 1989—the federal government's second major change in the Medicare system—Congress moved more definitively to assure the restraint of federal expenditures for physician services, which had increased threefold (in current dollars) over the decade.

One of the principal objectives of the new legislation was to rationalize economic incentives between physicians engaged primarily in cognitive treatment and surgeons and other proceduralists and to balance the outcome by increasing the earnings of the former and reducing those of the latter. In preparing the federal budget for 1992, the administration decided to adopt the newly formulated Resource Based Relative Value Scale (RBRVS) in order to realize substantial budgetary savings, but this decision precipitated a major struggle between the medical profession and the federal government over the future of the new legislation. In the viewpoint of the leaders of American medicine and Congress, the administration broke faith with the many medical societies that had helped to draft the legislation and assisted in getting it passed. In the face of this vehement opposition, the administration retreated.

At the end of the decade (in 1989), the federal government's share of national health expenditures was the same as it had been in 1980—29 percent. State and local governments also experienced no relative change in their share—they accounted for 13 percent at the start and at the end of the 1980s. The most significant shift was in the share of private health insurance which rose from 29 to 33 percent or by 14 percent. The increase was compensated by small percentage declines in out-of-pocket payments and payments from other private sources.

On its face, it is hard to explain this rise in the contribution of private health insurance in a period when the total number of workers with health benefits was declining, when a fair number of employers persuaded their workforces to agree to deductibles and coinsurance, and, most important, when virtually all large and many medium-sized employers resorted to ever more elaborate systems of managed care as a means of decelerating their health care costs. The best reconciliation between the efforts made by employers to contain their costs and the increasing share of the rapidly expanding total national outlays that devolved upon private insurance involves several factors. Many of the employers' cost-saving efforts yielded a one-time saving, such as the move of large corporations to self-insure. Many of their utilization control measures and their more elaborate managed-care initiatives produced only modest results. "Cost-shifting" also played a major role. In a multiple-payer system such as that prevailing in the United States, any shortfall by one or more of the payers—the federal government, state governments, or individuals—is shifted, if at all possible, by the providers to the residual payer(s), in this case, private health insurance. One informed estimate by students of hospital finance found that cost-shifting to private insurance by the hospitals amounted to $57 billion in 1990, over and above the $85 billion of full-cost reimbursement for services provided.

The early 1980s also saw heightened entrepreneurialism in the health sector: the peak expansion of for-profit hospital chains that began in the late 1960s and early 1970s; the continued proliferation of for-profit ambulatory care facilities (for primary care and minor surgery) and of specialized hospitals (psychiatric and substance-abuse); and old and new types of prepayment plans such as HMOs and preferred provider organizations (PPOs). It has been estimated that as a result of this across-the-board penetration by the for-profit sector, its share of total health care expenditures rose from 17 percent in 1979 to 21 percent in 1990.

Several facts about the rapidly advancing role of the for-profit sector are worth noting. The dramatic growth of the for-profit hospital chains was concentrated in a limited number of areas, primarily California and several states in the South and Southwest; they made little or no headway in other parts of the country for a variety of reasons, including (in New

York) outright legislative interdiction. It should also be emphasized that the growth of the chains (the largest were Hospital Corporation of America, Humana, American Medical International, and National Medical Enterprises) was nurtured by liberal federal and state reimbursement policies, which enabled them to earn a return on debt, capitalize depreciation, and, in particular, obtain a generous return on equity as well. What is more, several of the states in which the chains were strongly represented based reimbursement rates on charges, not audited costs.

When the for-profit chains were the darlings of Wall Street because of their dependable cash flows and consistent earnings growth of 20 percent or more per annum, some analysts and academicians propagated the doctrine that their exceptional track record reflected the superiority of their organizational and managerial skills over the capabilities of the traditional nonprofit hospitals. However, a close look at the evidence presented in support of this position revealed wide gaps in logic and analysis. Once the federal government shifted to a prospective payment system in 1983 and hospital admissions declined, the argument was settled definitively by the serious financial reverses of all of the major hospital chains.

The monetarization of the health care system was greatly accelerated by the passage of Medicare and Medicaid, which turned large numbers of charity patients into paying patients, and continued apace throughout the 1970s and the 1980s. Total outlays for health as a percentage of gross national product (GNP) rose from about 6.5 percent in 1965 to close to 12 percent in 1990. Nonprofit institutions, particularly large sophisticated hospitals that often had revenue flows of over $1 million a day, had little option but to become increasingly preoccupied with their competitive position in the marketplace and with their bottom line. Nonprofit or not, they were at risk unless their revenues consistently exceeded their expenditures, a condition necessary for them to obtain the capital funding they needed for continuous upgrading of their plants and equipment.

Among the important by-products of the growing financial exposure of the dominant nonprofit health institutions were their efforts, direct and indirect, to control the amount of free and below-cost care that they provided the poor and the near poor. A defensive strategy that some nonprofit hospitals adopted was to leave the inner-city location where they had long served large numbers of the neighborhood poor for suburban locations where their clientele would consist almost exclusively of well-insured persons. Others began to refer many uninsured patients to nearby or more distant public institutions. A number of nonprofit hospitals that were members of trauma networks experienced severe financial drains as a result of the high proportion of poorly insured or uninsured patients they were forced to admit for lengthy, costly treatment and withdrew from the networks. Some that were located in or near low-income neighborhoods closed their emergency rooms, which channeled many poor patients into the hospitals for definitive treatment. The identification of these practices and trends in the context of our earlier observations about the retrogression in the Medicaid program during the 1980s provides a concrete view of the worsening position of the poor and the uninsured in obtaining access to the health care system.

Compounding the deteriorating situation in the nonprofit sector, the funding of most public sector facilities—hospitals, clinics, child health stations, and the like—was also far below the amounts required to meet the increasing demands on them. And to complete the dismal picture, despite the growing number of graduates of American medical schools supplemented by the steady inflow of foreign medical graduates, the cadre of physicians able and willing to care for large or small concentrations of low-income urban and rural populations diminished rather than expanded, surely worsening their access to primary care. From area to area in many large cities, astronomical variations could be found in the ratio of private practitioners to population: An affluent neighborhood might have available 1 physician for 150 to 200 persons; in a low-income section, the ratio could be as low as 1 per 15,000.

The adoption by private insurance companies of aggressive risk-management techniques in the 1980s resulted in increasing difficulties for various groups to obtain or renew their health coverage at an affordable cost. The health insurance companies sought to reduce their risks by refusing to enroll or to renew insurance for persons with serious preexisting medical conditions, such as heart disease or cancer. They also quoted increasingly high rates to small employers so that many discontinued covering their workforce. A large number of insurance companies stopped writing individual policies altogether. In pursuing its profit-seeking objectives, the health insurance sector indirectly contributed to the undermining of the U.S. health care system by revoking the opportunities of millions of persons to obtain or renew private insurance coverage.

With the federal government focusing in the 1980s almost exclusively on efforts to moderate its steadily increasing expenditures for Medicare and to a lesser extent Medicaid, numerous initiatives were undertaken by the states in response to a wide range of health policy issues, from the introduction of competitive bidding by hospitals for authorization to admit Medicaid patients to the establishment of state-subsidized risk pools to enable individuals to obtain insurance coverage at prices they could afford. A few states obtained waivers from the federal government that permitted them to establish a single-payer system for hospital care. Others moved to enroll Medicaid beneficiaries in HMOs with an eye toward saving money and improving the quality of care available to them. A number established statewide pools to reimburse hospitals that provide disproportionate amounts of uncompensated care to indigent patients as a means of ensuring their continued operation.

The foregoing is a small sampling of the many initiatives that the states launched at different times during the 1980s; a considerable amount of experimentation continues today. But all of the experimentation that the states have attempted should not obscure the fact that their primary involvement in health care has been centered on the financing of Medicaid, a task that they have found increasingly onerous as a result of the growth in enrollment mandated by federal legislation and steadily rising costs.

By virtue of its unique function and responsibility for treating patients, the medical profession continued to play a critical role in the evolution of national health policy in the 1980s, although most members of the profession felt the lead had been wrested from them as their clinical decision-making authority was subjected to increasing surveillance. Prior permission from the payer became a requirement for admitting a patient to the hospital, for undertaking selected diagnostic or therapeutic interventions, and for retaining a patient in the hospital beyond a fixed number of days. What is more, many payers contested the fees that they were billed.

To make matters worse, the 1980s saw the continued growth of malpractice suits, which meant that in addition to facing higher insurance premiums (in the case of obstetricians and neurosurgeons these could exceed $100,000 annually), physicians found their relationships with patients strained because of the ever present threat of litigation. With their clinical judgments subject to second-guessing by nonphysician employees of payer organizations and with the trust relationship between physician and patient undermined, much of the gratification of medical practice was lost. It is not surprising that many medical students interviewed reported having been advised against applying to medical school by a large proportion of the physicians whom they had consulted about their career plans.

Despite these serious disincentives to medical practice in the 1980s, which led some physicians to decide on early retirement and others to limit their practice (for instance, a fair number of obstetricians-gynecologists stopped performing deliveries in an effort to reduce their malpractice liability), high-tech medicine continued to make significant strides as a consequence of breakthroughs in medical research and technique. Budgetary pressures notwithstanding, the two-term Reagan administration found the funds to enlarge the real expenditure levels for biomedical research and development (R&D), and at decade's end the federal contribution was in excess of $10 billion annually.

Even so, the acquired immune deficiency syndrome (AIDS) pandemic that came without forewarning found the basic scientists and the medical practitioners overwhelmed. Although the research community has been working overtime, primarily with belated federal funding, to develop an effective vaccine, the achievement of this goal is not imminent. To date, the most notable outcome has been the development of a few drugs that can attenuate the progress of the disease and postpone death for a period of months or years. The measures that the public must follow to avoid contracting the disease have also been identified and publicized, no small contribution to containing its damage potential.

Despite the enthusiasm of most physicians, political leaders and the public at large for high-tech medicine, a counterdevelopment emerged during the 1980s. Largely as a consequence of the work of Dr. John Wennberg of Dartmouth and the health policy research staff at RAND, a considerable amount of disturbing evidence was accumulated that raised serious questions about the efficacy of many widely used medical and surgical interventions. Although the evidence did not produce unequivocal answers as to which conventional practices were acceptable and which were not, it did underscore the need for more precise definitions and information concerning the "outcomes" of medical intervention if patients were not to be exposed to increasing risk and if valuable resources were not to be wasted.

By the end of the decade, Congress established a new office, the Agency for Health Care Policy and Research, with a reasonable amount of funding (circa $100 million) to take the lead in designing and carrying out valid outcome studies in the hope that these would lead both to an improved quality of care and to economies in resource use through the formulation and adoption of practice guidelines. The American Medical Association (AMA), RAND, and several academic health centers (AHCs) entered into a cooperative set of investigations.

At this early stage, high expectations are held for outcome studies, although some of the leading investigators, including Dr. Robert Brook of RAND, have warned that as far as economic gains are concerned, the expectations may not materialize. Clinical analyses may well find that the number of persons exposed to expensive, unneeded, and possibly contraindicated procedures is balanced or even outweighed by the number who could benefit from such procedures but are currently not receiving them and who should and would receive them in a better-controlled environment. Whatever the results, the odds strongly favor the 1990s being a decade of intensified outcomes research with the dual aim of improving the quality of health care and making more efficient use of health resources.

With the advantage of hindsight, we can summarize health care delivery in the 1980s as follows: The majority of well-insured Americans enjoyed access to a more sophisticated level of health care at the end than at the beginning of the period. The costs of operating the system mounted steeply, putting severe pressures on the three principal payers—the federal government, state governments, and employers. For one-third of the population—namely persons with shallow insurance, Medicaid enrollees, and the uninsured—access to health and hospital care, both preventive and therapeutic, deteriorated. Although a small number of rural and inner-city hospitals failed, the vast majority came through the trying decade with a positive margin; at the beginning of the 1990s, however, a not inconsiderable number—between 15 and 20 percent—are nearing or have entered the danger zone.

During the 1980s, physicians' earnings not only remained high, absolutely and relative to other groups in the population, but in fact improved. However, the environment of medical practice deteriorated as a result of the physicians' loss both of clinical freedom and of the respect and confidence of their patients and, more particularly, of the public at large.

Various leadership groups, voluntary and governmental, addressed the issues of U.S. health system reform during the decade, but their findings and recommendations failed to capture the imagination and support either of the public or of its political leaders. As a consequence, no major efforts at reform were initiated, let alone carried out. The single federal effort, legislation passed in 1988 to provide catastrophic benefits under Medicare, was rescinded the following year in response to a revolt of affluent Medicare beneficiaries who objected to paying higher taxes to finance the new, enhanced benefits. With the exception of the serious erosion in the ability of the poor and the uninsured to obtain access to health care services, the decade of the 1980s ended as it had begun—with a substantial legacy of long-standing problems and solutions still to be found.

The activities of the national administration and Congress during the fifteen years between the passage of Medicare and the election of Ronald Reagan demonstrated that for a variety of reasons the federal government was no longer inclined to exercise a leadership role in the reform of the U.S. health care system, and as the 1980s progressed this stance was reinforced. The federal government's concerns were directed first and foremost at moderating its outlays for health care; yet its repeated efforts to do so, following a variety of approaches, produced limited results at best.

Once the federal government yielded its long-held place as innovator and reformer of the nation's health care system, it was inevitable in our federal-state system that the states would be catapulted into positions of greater prominence in the shaping of health policy. Hence a shift in the focus of policy research to state priorities and actions was indicated together with a corresponding redirection of inquiries into the institutional structure and operations of the system. Because the delivery of medical care is conditioned by the patient's place of residence, by the location and quality of hospital and ambulatory facilities, and by the preferences of physicians and other health care personnel with respect to their mode and location of practice, it was obvious that the unit of investigation should be the medical infrastructure in place in different geographic areas.

Accordingly, in 1986 the Eisenhower Center staff proposed to The Robert Wood Johnson Foundation, the sponsor of much of its earlier health policy research, a three-year monitoring study of the changing health care delivery systems in the nation's four largest metropolitan centers—New York, Chicago, Houston, and Los Angeles. Their four parent states—New York, Illinois, Texas, and California—represented four major regions of the country, and together they accounted for 74 million persons, or roughly one third of the nation's population. These metropolitan areas differed in many respects, including their historical background, demographic profile, racial composition, and philanthropic structure; the role of the public sector in health care delivery; the presence of AHCs; and other critical dimensions affecting the demand, supply, and financing of health care services. Moreover, the health care policies of the four parent states differed substantially in terms of such critical issues as their preference for regulation or competition; the nature (liberal or restrictive) of their Medicaid programs; their reimbursement policies; and other state-specific factors. Basic structural and operational differences included the relative importance of HMOs and other alternative delivery systems; hospital occupancy rates; the scope, influence, and vitality of the for-profit sector; the governance of the public sector; and the adequacy and mix of health care personnel.

The study aimed to delineate the specific developments within each metro and to capture and analyze the differences and the parallels among the four that might illuminate the dynamics and the contours of change in the nation's health care system. In justification of this subnational approach, the proposal noted that the macroforecasting techniques conventionally utilized for delineating the future shape of health care delivery in the U.S. had severe limitations, among them:

- The difficulty of making reasonable assumptions about the economic parameters (including the rate of growth of the U.S. economy; the timing, severity, and length of the next recession; productivity trends; and so forth) that would help to determine societal demands and resources
- The profound implications of unforeseeable changes in the economic environment for investment and utilization patterns in the health care sector

- The differential impact of macroeconomic factors upon specific components of the extant system of care, as, for instance, the ease or difficulty of financing the care of the poor as compared to the financing of AHCs.

The proposed subnational level of analysis was designed to accomplish three tasks: to establish a baseline profile of the health care system in each of the four metros; to identify the more potent elements of change that were operating locally and regionally, and to assess the interactions between the extant system and the most potent change agents.

Among the areas selected for investigation were the following:

- Alternative responses to the growing surplus of acute-care hospital beds
- The potentiators of, and the impediments to, the expansion of HMOs and other innovative forms of health care delivery
- Public and private responses to the uncompensated-care issue
- The establishment of new ambulatory-care facilities—diagnostic, therapeutic, and rehabilitative—and their interaction with the existing hospitals
- The responses of both the governmental and nongovernmental sectors to the growing surplus of physicians and the supply of other health care personnel
- The impact of pressures imposed by declining hospital admissions and early discharges on the nursing home and home health care sectors
- The principal consequences for local AHCs of the more price-competitive environment and the shift from inpatient to ambulatory treatment
- The degree of satisfaction/disappointment among the local business coalitions with progress toward their major goals and the modification of those goals with experience
- Identification of the health care issues that commanded the attention of the press, the public, and political groups and the actions taken in response to them

It was recognized at the outset that this subnational research design could not be effectively implemented in so dynamic a sector of the economy as medical care by centralized investigators distant from the field of operations. Data gathering and first-order analysis required the collaboration of resident researchers in the four metros who were well acquainted with the operation of the health care system in their respective locales and who were willing to participate in a joint assessment of ongoing changes for the period of study, 1987-1989, through the use of a structured monitoring protocol. The success of the undertaking was dependent on the identification of three principal collaborators—in Chicago, Los Angeles, and Houston. The Eisenhower Center staff assumed responsibility for the New York City study.

As is not infrequently the case, the research design underwent an important modification soon after the project got under way. The proposal had originally included the establishment of a baseline profile of the health care system in each of the metros as of 1985—that is, just prior to the start of the monitoring period. However, developing such a recent baseline proved neither feasible nor desirable. The longer perspective of the health care system in each of the metros as it was operating at the beginning of the 1980s was needed in order to judge more incisively and more confidently the changes actually under way and the forces responsible for them. With this lengthened perspective, the investigators were better positioned to identify the parallels and differences in the medical infrastructures of the four sites from the vantage point of such · basics as medical institutions, health delivery systems, and politics, all of which, by virtue of the forces of inertia, were likely to provide important elements of continuity even in a decade of significant change. As the research progressed, it became evident that the scheme needed to be broadened to accommodate not only the ways in which metropolitan-state developments were altering the structure and functioning of the health care system but also the impact of new national, governmental, and market forces.

Coincidentally, in 1988 The Commonwealth Fund awarded a major grant, in which the Eisenhower Center participated, for a special inquiry into the nursing shortage. Surveys of nurse supply and demand were conducted in six major cities, among them the four metros that are the subject of this study. The overlap of the two studies was felicitous in that it provided additional data and insights regarding health system changes in these four sites particularly as they related to hospital operations.

The reader must judge whether the state-local focus of this work was justified by what it has succeeded in uncovering about the changing contours of the health delivery system in the nation's four largest urban centers during the 1980s. The dynamism of health care during the decade, as the proposal hypothesized, received its major impetus not from the federal government but rather from the forces that determined local demand for health care services and from the ability and willingness of the individual health care systems to respond to new needs and new public priorities.

Bibliography

Coddington, D.C., *The Crisis in Health Care: Costs, Choices, and Strategies* (San Francisco: Jossey-Bass, 1990).

Relman, A.S., Shattuck Lecture—"The Health Care Industry: Where Is It Taking Us?" *The New England Journal of Medicine* 325 (12): (September 19, 1991): 854–859.

Russell, L., *Medicare's New Hospital Payment System: Is It Working?* (Washington, D.C.: The Brookings Institution, 1989).

2

Changes in the Health Care Delivery System in New York City: 1980–1990

Howard S. Berliner

Demographics and Economics

New York City is, with a population of over 7.2 million residents reported in the 1980 census, still the largest city in the United States, notwithstanding a substantial drop from the 8 million residents counted in 1960. Although, the 1990 census results have been challenged for their accuracy, they currently show some growth over 1980. The most noticeable change between 1980 and 1990 was the increase in the minority population, particularly the black, Hispanic, and Asian groups. Especially significant were the increases in the number of people living in poverty and in the number who were homeless. It is difficult to find a valid estimate of the number of illegal aliens, often placed at between 500,000 and 750,000, but certainly they constituted a substantial segment of the population.

An examination of the city's economy during the 1980s must first look to the fiscal crisis of 1975 and its impact on both New York City and New York State. The near bankruptcy of the city caused the city government to lay off large numbers of municipal workers and to pare the municipal budget—a process that hit the health sector particularly hard. Although New York City climbed back to a period of relative fiscal health by the mid-1980s, most services had not been restored to prefiscal crisis staffing or budget levels. Over the study period (1980–1990), the economy of the city continued to shift from its historical base of light industry and manufacture toward the provision of services. For the health system the impact of this change lay primarily in fewer people having health insurance coverage. The service economy is not a stable one, and the effects of the Wall Street crash of 1987 and the more recent quasi-crash of 1989 are stark illustrations of just how sensitive the urban economy is to major fluctuations in the stock market. Whereas unemployment rates were below the national average (although not below the regional average) at the end of the decade, the quality of the jobs available, in terms of income and benefits, was questionable. Masked by the low unemployment rates was the fact that labor force participation rates were also consistently low. Despite the changes in the demographics and the economy of the city, the welfare rolls remained relatively stable, although some upturn was seen as the recession began to take its toll by early 1990. This stability seems to have been a function of the careful administrative rationing of benefits.

The Acute-Care System

Table 2.1 reveals that the major changes in the acute-care infrastructure took place in the period between 1975 and 1980 and that there was relatively little structural change after 1980. No new acute-care beds were added in New York City between 1975 and 1988. Faced with having to pay increasing reimbursements to hospitals with only average occupancy, the State Department of Health began a campaign to close what were perceived to be surplus acute-care beds. The strategy involved imposing severe reimbursement penalties on hospitals with under 85 percent occupancy as an incentive to increase admissions or close beds and encouraging, if not forcing, the closure, merger, or reduction of acute-care services and facilities. In view of the decreased number of beds, it is not surprising that occupancy rates rose. Although admissions fell slightly, they did not keep pace with the declining inpatient capacity.

Not reflected in the aggregated hospital utilization statistics are the occupancy and emergency room crises of 1988 and 1989. Changes in the state reimbursement policy that further increased penalties for hospitals operating at less than 90 percent occupancy were instituted in 1988. To avoid these penalties hospitals were forced to declare large numbers of acute-care beds out of service on January 1, 1989, and as a result, occupancy rates were artificially inflated to over 90 percent in most hospitals. The media picked up on this "occupancy crisis" and blamed it on the increasing number of AIDS, substance-abusing, mentally ill, and homeless patients being treated in hospitals. Although it is certainly true that these social pathologies were not anticipated and were not factored into health planning needs assessments and projections, it is also true that state and local health planners were operating under strict orders to decrease acute-care capacity independent of any objective reality. The acute-care occupancy problems were due as much to such factors as staffing shortages, which necessitated closing beds and units in hospitals, and intentional backlogs of emergency rooms to limit the number of indigent patients ad-

TABLE 2.1   Hospital Capacity and Utilization, New York City, 1975, 1980, and 1989

	1975	*1980*	*1989*
Number of hospitals			
Voluntary	67	56	53
Public	18	13	11
Proprietary	31	16	14
Total	116	85	78
Number of acute-care beds			
Voluntary	25,332	23,978	22,622
Public	8,108	6,629	5,687
Proprietary	4,274	2,687	1,727
Total	37,714	33,294	30,036
Occupancy (percent)			
Voluntary	89.2	84.4	88.7
Public	74.5	80.8	83.9
Proprietary	83.4	82.8	81.5
Total	82.4	82.7	86.4
Average length of stay (days)			
Voluntary	10.8	9.5	8.7
Public	10.9	10.2	8.9
Proprietary	8.6	7.8	7.5
Total	10.1	9.2	8.4

Source: Health Systems Agency of New York City, Community Health Profiles, 1991.

mitted as to the new populations seeking care. Emergency room and outpatient department (OPD) volumes have increased in recent years, but this increase must be assessed in the context of the historically high usage of institutional outpatient services in New York City. Anecdotally, the major change confronting the emergency room in the 1980s was not a sudden influx of population so much as a change in the population seeking care. The large number of trauma patients (gunshot wounds, stabbings, etc.) occupied the attention of staff and caused major backlogs for patients with less severe problems. In addition, shortages of critical-care nurses, in an era of high negligence litigation, forced hospitals to close intensive care beds at a time when they were most needed. With intensive care units (ICUs) operating at reduced levels, emergency rooms were less able to accept new patients, and thus backlogs began to grow. Interestingly, the media in New York soured on this story by early 1989 and have devoted little attention to it since that time, although in quantitative terms the backlogs have gotten worse.

Academic Medical Centers in New York City

New York City is distinguished by the fact that virtually all of its hospitals are teaching hospitals. Thirty hospitals are members of the Council of Teaching Hospitals (COTH). There are six medical schools located within city limits; a seventh, which relocated some years ago to a suburban county to the north, still maintains a large number of teaching hospitals in the city. Nine of the eleven public acute-care hospitals in New York City are affiliated with either medical schools or the voluntary hospitals that serve as their major teaching facilities. The other nonteaching institutions are mainly small proprietary hospitals located in the outer boroughs, institutions that will probably not survive the early 1990s.

State policy has encouraged the establishment of teaching and referral relations between AHCs and community hospitals as a mechanism for ensuring the quality of care at the community hospitals and for controlling and moderating access to new technologies. Thus, as a condition for certificate of need (CON) approval of major modernization and rebuilding programs by the AHCs in Manhattan, the state required those institutions to provide financial, technical, and medical support to small voluntary hospitals.

State approval for hospitals to provide new high-technology services in New York City—such as imaging, transplants, and lithotripsy—is first given to the AHCs, which are charged with establishing consortia of referral hospitals that will share in the use of the equipment or procedures. This de facto regionalization of services in New York City has not been very effective because the limitation of new technology by the state applies only to hospitals. New high-technology services remain available to physicians and entrepreneurs, independent of the strict regulatory system that controls hospitals. Thus, when there was only one CON-approved magnetic resonance imaging (MRI) scanner at an AHC in New York City, four others were already operating under private auspices—three owned by physician groups and one owned by an entrepreneur and leased to a physician group.

During the course of the study several AHCs underwent major modernization. Four of the six university teaching hospitals in the city underwent or are undergoing such major capital projects. For three of them (Presbyterian Hospital, Mount Sinai, and St. Luke's–Roosevelt), the cost came to almost $1.5 billion, and the cost incurred by the fourth (Montefiore) came to almost $250 million. In 1990, New York Hospital was preparing for a major modernization program, but it had to be delayed for financial reasons. The capital improvements were deemed necessary not only because the facilities were antiquated and inefficient but as a means for ensuring the viability of the urban medical centers and reducing their vulnerability to competition from suburban facilities.

Institutional Changes

As noted earlier in this chapter, most of the changes undergone by the hospital sector in New York City occurred in the years between 1975 and

1980. In this period the state greatly increased its authority over reimbursements and new hospital construction. Two new facilities were
opened, Woodhull Hospital and the Allen Pavilion. The first, Woodhull, is
a public hospital that was built in the early 1970s but due to the fiscal crisis
of the city at that time it did not commence operations until 1981 at the
same time that two older public hospitals closed. The second, Allen Pavilion, is a 300-bed community hospital located on the northern tip of Manhattan and affiliated with Presbyterian Hospital. It began to admit patients in 1988, replacing several small hospitals that had previously been
shut. Over the ten-year period virtually the entire hospital plant in the
City underwent some modernization. The hospitals in Brooklyn were significantly improved in the late 1970s and early 1980s as the result of a coordinated state plan; Manhattan and Bronx hospitals followed suit in the
mid- to late 1980s. In the early 1980s there was some hospital merger and
system formation activity, primarily in the outer boroughs. The Archdiocese of New York and the Archdiocese of Brooklyn formed networks and
systems for their institutions in their respective sees. Because an effective
joint purchasing service was already in operation under the auspices of
the Greater New York Hospital Association, there was little need for metropolitan hospitals to organize specifically for this task. Some of the larger
institutions joined Voluntary Hospitals of America (VHA), including New
York Hospital and Presbyterian Hospital, but their membership in the system seems to have been a strategic move with no practical consequences,
and they have since withdrawn. Planners at these hospitals reasoned that
the costs of joining a system such as VHA were relatively low and if the
systems proved to be useful in drawing new patients through their PPOs,
the hospitals would stand to gain considerably. As it turned out, the VHA
PPO was not successful in the New York area, and the hospitals did not
get any advantage out of the system. In general, multi-institutionalization
has not been a strategic option for New York City hospitals; their large
size limits the potential gains from economies of scale. Thus the hospitals
in New York already had many of the benefits that hospitals in other cities
obtained through joining systems or networks.

New York State law prohibits the establishment of investor-owned hospitals. As a result, New York City has had no experience with the phenomenon of proprietary hospital chains. The proprietary hospitals that exist in
the city are all individually owned.

Patient and Payer Mix

Changes in patient and payer mix in New York City hospitals have
been significant. For one thing, the number of nonresident patients utilizing New York City hospitals fell during the decade. In 1980 approximately
14 percent of the inpatients admitted to New York City hospitals lived

outside the borders of the city; by 1988, the number had declined to approximately 10 percent. Because most of these were charge-paying patients, the loss was significant and was exacerbated by the fact that these patients were probably replaced by nonpaying ones. Border hospitals were affected more severely than other hospitals in the city.

The percentage of patients who are enrolled in HMOs increased slightly over the decade, and this trend bears some explanation. The Health Insurance Plan (HIP), for a long time the only HMO-type organization in New York City, initially covered only ambulatory care, and its members purchased other private policies for inpatient care. However, HIP has been shifting to a more traditional type HMO and has been somewhat successful in reducing the hospital admissions of its members. With the addition of new HMOs that have sprung up around the metropolitan area, the net impact has been a decrease in the number of admissions to New York City hospitals.

During the 1980s the number of Medicaid patients remained fairly stable (in the 1.2–1.4 million range) in New York City. However, the number of uninsured patients increased considerably—to over 19 percent of the population. All hospitals in New York City accept Medicaid. Since 1981, when the first all-payer reimbursement system went into effect, hospitals have been reimbursed for their inpatient uncompensated care (though not at 100 percent). New York hospitals were thus among the first in the country to receive payment for the uninsured, and this payment, combined with the large number of publicly supported facilities, has given hospitals in the area the ability to take care of the indigent. Historically, there has been a tradition of private hospitals referring indigent and Medicaid patients to nearby (or physically connected) public hospitals. The hospitals with the worst financial problems in New York today are those without nearby public institutions that can admit indigent and Medicaid patients. Such hospitals include Presbyterian in Manhattan and Brookdale and Lutheran in Brooklyn.

Finances

The acute care hospitals in New York City lost over $400 million in 1990. A similar amount was lost in 1989, and aggregate losses of a smaller magnitude were experienced during the earlier part of the decade. During the 1980s, the operating margins of New York City hospitals declined from being marginally positive to negative. At the end of the decade overall margins were still positive for some institutions, but they had decreased. What is paradoxical about this situation is that the hospitals are not so much suffering from a shortage of patients as from a surplus of nonpaying patients, expensive operating costs, and expensive new technology. New York City hospitals provide large amounts of ambulatory and emergency care, for which they are not reimbursed at cost. The all-inclusive clinic visit fee of $60 that Medicaid pays hospitals has not been raised since the early 1980s, and even then it was seen as being below true cost. Because outpatient services are not fully reimbursed under the New York bad debt and charity care pools (except for services provided by financially distressed hospitals), and the bulk of services that are provided is either totally uncompensated or reimbursed at below cost, they have been the major reason for hospital financial problems. Most people utilizing outpatient services are either uninsured or on Medicaid. Blue Cross does not pay for outpatient services, and most other insurance plans assume that outpatient visits will be paid by the patient; therefore there is greater bad debt on the outpatient side than on the inpatient side of the hospital. Although hospitals have appealed to the state to raise the rate it pays for outpatient services, the state has declined for two basic reasons: (1) it wants to encourage hospitals to get rid of expensive hospital-based ambulatory care in favor of cheaper community primary care; and (2) raising the rate to a more reasonable level would cost too much. Increasing the rate to $100 per visit would require $300 million in new state revenues. Moreover, the high level of debt that many of the larger hospitals have accrued for modernization campaigns has forced hospitals to raise charges to patients who could not pay even the former, lower amounts.

Through much of the 1980s, New York State had a waiver from Medicare. PPS did not start in New York until January 1986, and when it did start, it was part of a reimbursement system that used DRGs for all payers (though they differ from those PPS uses). The impact of PPS was thus quite limited. New York City hospitals have always had one of the highest lengths of stay in the nation, and it seems that the average length of stay (ALOS) has increased with an all-DRG system. Although admissions of persons over sixty-five years of age have fallen, they have been made up by significant increases in admissions of those under sixty-five, primarily for AIDS, drug abuse, and mental health.

It appears that the main reason New York City hospitals sought to eliminate the Medicare waiver was that without the waiver they would have a second source of revenue that would be outside the control of the state health department. Although initial projections of how much more the hospitals would receive from PPS than from the state formula looked quite promising, it was clear to all observers that the PPS reimbursement would soon be cut and perhaps would be cut back well below what New York State was paying. PPS did not reimburse in full for capital, the allowance for graduate medical education (GME) was cut back, and was barely covering inflationary increases, let alone new technology. At the same time, upstate hospitals seemed to have significantly more to gain from PPS than the downstate (New York City) hospitals did. It is too soon to as-

sess whether ending the waiver was a smart strategic move on the part of
the hospitals, but certainly the hospitals traded a greater ability to influence rate changes for a weaker influence on the federal level. Upstate hospitals have done relatively well. Their profit margins are not high, but
they are far better than those for downstate institutions because of the far
lower number of Medicaid and uninsured patients they admit.

Emergency Services

New York State requires every hospital to operate an emergency room.
In New York City the emergency medical system (EMS) is run by the
Health and Hospitals Corporation. Until recently, hospitals had the option
of becoming receiving hospitals or opting out of the system. Before 1986,
many of the larger medical centers in New York City, including Mount Sinai, New York Hospital, and New York University Hospital, were not receiving hospitals in the emergency medical system. State pressure has
since forced these hospitals into the system.

There are three separate emergency medical systems in New York: (1)
the 911 system; (2) voluntary, community-based ambulance systems; and
(3) private ambulance systems. The 1980s were marked by the inability to
get these three systems to cooperate in even the most basic ways. An even
more serious problem was the reluctance of voluntary hospitals to receive
patients via the emergency room for fear that they would turn out to be
uninsured and in need of large amounts of care. The hospitals were primarily concerned that trauma cases entering via the emergency room
would tie up operating suites and intensive care units and would thus not
allow them to admit paying elective surgery patients. As a result, each
winter there has been an ambulance diversion crisis that has lasted until
occupancy rates began their normal decline as warmer weather ap-
proached. Voluntary hospitals commonly remove themselves from the receiving hospital system for each shift, claiming that their emergency
rooms are tied up or that their intensive care units are filled. Ambulances
are forced to travel around the city until they can find a hospital that will
allow them to drop off a patient. These issues have not been resolved, nor
are they likely to be resolved in the near future. During the winter of
1988-1989 emergency rooms (ERs) throughout the city were filled well beyond capacity, and patients were kept in ERs for long periods of time.
Consequently, state regulations went into effect in January 1989 mandating that patients could stay no more than eight hours in an emergency
room without being admitted. The regulation did not address what would
happen if they could not be admitted. The ER crowding problem did not
seem to be as bad in 1989, but few observers attribute this fact to the regulations; the trend may reflect a decrease in media coverage rather than any
significant change in the situation.

Hospitals in New York City accommodated over 11 million outpatient and ER visits in 1989 (7.8 million outpatient and 3.2 million ER). Clinics in the larger hospitals registered as many as 650,000 visits per year. Community health centers at their peak (1982) provided another million visits in thirty-two sites. The number of community health centers declined over the decade to only sixteen; they provided some 350,000 visits in 1989.

Diversification Strategies

During the 1980s, New York City's demarketing became a more attractive strategy to voluntary hospitals than marketing and continues to be so. The many possible sources of marketing for new patients were not aggressively explored, international patients, tourists, patients from the suburbs, and patients from outlying areas were all left largely to their own devices. Instead, hospitals concentrated their efforts at trying to get rid of patients whom they did not want. These demarketing strategies included closing some outpatient clinics, limiting outpatient services to residents of narrowly defined catchment areas, and referring patients to public hospitals.

Mount Sinai Hospital and to a lesser extent St. Luke's–Roosevelt and Beth Israel engaged in extensive marketing of their services in New York City. St. Luke's and Beth Israel advertised their physician referral services, but only Mount Sinai undertook a multimedia campaign to attract patients. Manhattan medical centers revealed a marked lack of interest in the possibility of attracting more foreign and out-of-town patients in a more organized manner than they currently do. New York City hospitals have been hurt by the loss of patients coming from surrounding areas—particularly, New Jersey, Westchester County and Long Island. These communities have established and elaborated local medical facilities, and patients from those areas no longer feel the need to go to New York City for treatment. The inconveniences of the city—parking difficulties, busy traffic to and from the hospitals, the fear of street crime, and the city's old and unappealing hospital facilities—have not helped.

There was little horizontal integration among hospitals in New York City, except for some hospital mergers in the outer boroughs. Forward vertical integration was attempted more frequently, and at the end of the decade a number of hospitals operated home health care services. There were few examples of backward integration. No new inpatient psychiatric or rehabilitation services were established in this period.

Public Hospitals

The New York City Health and Hospitals Corporation (HHC) is a quasi-public agency, with a majority of its board of directors appointed by the mayor of New York City. Hospitals belonging to HHC have a statutory responsibility to accept all patients regardless of their ability to pay, and the corporation's deficit is made up from city tax levy funds. Throughout the 1980s efforts were made to increase the level of third-party reimbursement that HHC hospitals received, but the success of these efforts were met with corresponding decreases in the level of funding from the city. The statewide bad debt and charity care pool discriminates against public hospitals in New York City in order to force the city to maintain its commitment.

The clientele of HHC hospitals changed appreciably over the decade, primarily with the great increase in the number of AIDS patients, mentally ill patients, the homeless, and substance abusers. Although large numbers of these patients were also treated at the city's voluntary hospitals, the increase was far greater in the public sector. The socioeconomic status of the patients decreased as the overall level of poverty in New York City increased over the decade.

The mission statement adopted by the HHC in 1990 recognizes that the system serves as the family doctor to the majority of its patients and as such must meet their needs through expanded primary and ambulatory-care services. At the same time, HHC has made the commitment to guarantee high technology and subspecialty services to the patients who utilize its facilities. As a result, HHC hospitals have aggressively pursued the acquisition of high technology (or made contractual arrangements with voluntary hospitals to ensure access to such services for their patients) while simultaneously trying to expand their ability to deliver primary care. Several arrangements have been made for HHC patients to utilize high-technology services not available at public facilities. Thus, Bellevue Hospital has arranged to utilize the radiation therapy services of New York University Hospital, and two public hospitals in the Bronx have worked out arrangements to regionalize ophthalmic services with two private hospitals located nearby. Patients at Queens Hospital Center needing cardiac catheterization are sent by arrangement to Long Island Jewish Hospital.

Of the eleven public hospitals in New York City, three underwent major modernization/renovation in the 1970s; five were modernized/renovated in the 1960s; and three have not had extensive renovation since the 1950s. Although capital plans have been made to continue the modernization process in hospitals throughout the city and to replace the obsolete Kings County Hospital plant with a new facility, financial considerations have forced the postponement of the major projects. The Kings County project, currently estimated to cost over $1 billion, has been delayed by a combination of factors, but the most important is the inability to raise the funds. It had been assumed that a Federal Housing Administration (FHA) loan could be obtained to meet the costs of the project, but the Reagan administration was not willing to invest much money in a New York City public hospital, and there is no evidence that the Bush administration will alter that position. At the same time, New York State has been seeking to unload the Downstate University Hospital, which it carries as a state budget line item, and spin it off as a voluntary facility. It would like to combine the facility with a new Kings County Hospital—a prospect that has been fought by both the HHC and the State University of New York (SUNY) Downstate Medical School. Finally, the rebuilding of Kings County Hospital will mean the rationalization of a very decentralized institution and the elimination of a large number of patronage jobs that were maintained under the old arrangements. This has not helped to facilitate the project.

All of the HHC facilities were downsized over the course of the decade either to avoid occupancy-related reimbursement penalties or because staff shortages forced bed closures. At the same time, HHC enhanced its ability to provide ambulatory care by increasing the number of hospital-affiliated primary care centers and neighborhood family care centers that it operates. Yet the demand for acute-care services at the public hospitals remained high at the end of the decade, particularly in those areas where the hospitals were the sole providers of care.

For the most part, HHC facilities are located in or near concentrations of medical indigence in New York. Two areas of Manhattan (the Lower East Side and Washington Heights/Inwood) are poverty centers that no longer have public facilities. In both of those areas, public hospitals were closed during the 1970s. There are large medically indigent populations in eastern Brooklyn and south Jamaica, Queens, for whom public hospitals are not readily accessible. These indigent populations use the large ambulatory-care facilities (neighborhood family care centers or community health centers) or the local voluntary hospitals or they travel to find a public hospital. The long waits for clinic visits imply a lack of provisions for primary and preventive service.

The public hospital system is widely thought to provide lower quality care than private hospitals. There are some notable centers of excellence—trauma care, microsurgery, the nurse-midwife program at North Central Bronx (NCB) Hospital, the acupuncture center at Lincoln Hospital—but for public hospitals overall, the quality of care is not considered to be high. The common perception, which is generally true, is that the hospitals are understaffed, operate with obsolete or broken equipment, and do not function with a high level of competence. Although the central administration of the HHC has been able to improve its public perception and hence its ability to lobby and raise money for its member hospitals, it was able to do so more because a former president of HHC became the deputy mayor responsible for human services than because of any dramatic change in performance.

Public hospitals accommodated 1.2 million (37.6 percent) of the 3.2 million emergency room visits in New York City in 1989. In the same year, they accommodated 3.8 million (48.8 percent) of the 7.8 million total outpatient department visits.

Summary

Hospitals in New York City did not seem much different at the end of the decade than they did at the start. The hospitals remained large, stodgy, inert institutions with little reason or incentive to change their current practices. They had not, except in very specific cases, made any of the changes that other hospitals around the country had been making. At the same time, it must be noted that they had not made as many mistakes as other hospitals around the country had made by getting involved in areas where they had no expertise or too little capital to develop a new base of operations. In short, they "stuck to the knitting," with all the limitations and benefits that such a strategy brings. One reason they adopted this strategy was their financial decline, which had limited their ability to pursue new approaches and new ventures even if they wanted to get involved. Although the New York State reimbursement system paid hospitals for a portion of their charity care and bad debt, it under-reimbursed for outpatient and emergency room services and it did not allow hospitals to shift costs onto other payers. As a result, hospitals were forced to spend capital and nonoperating funds to make up operational deficits caused by ambulatory services. Changes in health insurance policies that promoted ambulatory surgery took business away from hospitals, and the tight regulatory system limited the revenues they could generate through the acquisition of new technology. The all-payer system diminished any incentive they might have had to explore new ventures because, with this system, their potential revenues were limited by formula. Hospitals would also point out the change in the nature of the patients that they had to care for and the meagerness of the reimbursement formula. Indisputably, the hospitals of New York City were in worse financial shape at the end of the decade then they were at the beginning.

Long-Term Care

The significant developments in long-term care in New York City in the 1980s include the growth of home care, the introduction of a case intensity reimbursement methodology based on resource utilization groups (RUGS) to control nursing home costs and to redress discriminatory admission policies, and a persistent shortage of nursing home facilities and beds.

Home care initially grew in New York as a method for reducing Medicaid institutional long-term care costs through the Nursing Home Without Walls program, which started in the late 1970s. In an attempt to stimulate the growth of home care services in New York, legislation was passed in the early 1980s that allowed for-profit (investor-owned) home care services to be established in the state. Many such firms entered the New York market, and although the more traditional home care agencies (e.g., the visiting nurse associations [VNAs]) controlled the bulk of basic home care, the for-profit firms did establish their niche in high-tech home care and specialty services. In 1988, New York City spent 63 percent of all the Medicaid money in the United States devoted to home care. By the end of the decade, the New York City program covered approximately 50,000 people at a cost of over $1 billion yearly. Yet, home care programs remained far cheaper than institutional long-term care because the wages of home care workers remained minimal. Any increase in those wages would have significantly increased the costs of the program. It has been estimated that each one cent per hour wage increase translates into $1 million in program cost; thus a raise of $1.00 per hour would add $100 million to the cost of the program.

Due to a significant differential in reimbursement, nursing homes in New York in the early 1980s sought to be classified as skilled nursing facilities (SNF) rather than health related facilities (HRF). Once the units were so classified, they attempted to restrict admissions to the least sick patients because the reimbursement was the same regardless of the health of the patients and the costs of caring for healthier patients were lower. As a result, the state instituted its resource utilization groups (RUGS) in 1984, essentially a DRG-type system for classifying patients for whom facilities were reimbursed. Since that time, there has been less concern about nursing home reimbursement on the part of administrators, and it has been somewhat easier for patients to get into nursing homes despite their condition.

Although there is a clear need for many more nursing home beds than are currently available, the state has effectively limited new construction by placing constraints on allowable capital reimbursement costs. The ceiling cost of a new nursing home bed in 1990 is $70,000, an amount well below the estimated $120,000 required to build a nursing home bed in New York City. Given the high costs of real estate in New York and the high building costs, new construction virtually ground to a halt over the decade. State estimates put the need for new nursing home beds at over 2,500, and industry sources estimate that 5,000 is closer to reality, but both of these estimates are based on formulas that are intentionally weighted to keep the need projections low.

Ambulatory Care

Table 2.2 shows recent enrollment numbers for metropolitan area HMOs. No comparable figures are available for PPOs. There are no officially licensed ambulatory surgery centers in New York City and only a handful of individually owned walk-in clinics, which differ little from private practices. There are no primary care center chains or other organized proprietary ambulatory-care sites. The alternative delivery systems in New York City have clearly not experienced rapid growth. As the table illustrates, most of the alternative delivery systems in New York are oriented toward the suburbs of the metropolis, and if the enrollments could be further analyzed, it is likely that they would reveal that the majority of the city membership is in the outer boroughs rather than in Manhattan. State law permitting the establishment of for-profit HMOs was enacted in New York in 1984. State legislators who observed the successful growth of home care services after proprietary firms were allowed into the market reasoned that HMO growth could be fostered and that ensuing health care costs would be lower if HMOs were allowed to compete for business in New York. However, land and construction costs in New York City made the capitalization of new clinics prohibitive, and the dearth of large group practices, particularly in primary care fields, required substantial contracting with individual physicians and the adoption of individual practice association (IPA) models of practice to provide services to subscribers.

The first major push came from Maxicare, which created a subsidiary firm in New York City with equity contributions from several major teaching hospitals (Montefiore, Mount Sinai, Beth Israel, Maimonides, and Long Island Jewish, earning it the sobriquet Koshercare) and later expanded to include Presbyterian Hospital and some others. Each hospital agreed to encourage its physician staff to join the Maxicare physician groups. Thus the approach that Maxicare took was to be a high-quality provider of ambulatory services by linking with the major teaching hospitals of the city. Other HMOs took different tacks—Sanus Corporation developed contracts with hospitals and family physicians in the outer boroughs and assumed that it could garner enough business to force Manhattan specialists to discount their prices. This approach, known as the bridge and tunnel strategy, assumed that the resident population of Manhattan (1.2 million people) consisted largely of the poor and indigent and the extremely rich—neither group a good prospect for HMOs. U.S. Healthcare tried a blanketing approach over the entire metropolitan area. By the end of the decade, HMOs had not cracked the New York City market, and many of the companies abandoned the city. It should also be noted that Blue Cross established an IPA that took much of whatever new business was generated for the HMOs and that HIP, the large half-century old HMO of the City, benefited from the advertising and marketing done

TABLE 2.2   HMO Growth in the New York Metropolitan Area, 1987–1990

Name	City Enrollment 1987	City Enrollment 1990	Metro Area Enrollment 1987	Metro Area Enrollment 1990
HIP	710,256	735,837	897,368	899,356
BC/BS	44,290	77,507	69,488	139,055
US Health	18,976	80,790	48,356	165,715
Total Health	3,000	35,487	2,500	123,584
Oxford	6,000	59,000	14,100	64,000
Sanus	0	25,575	1,400	47,598
Travellers	3,000	39,000	7,000	107,900
MetLife	0	18,700	0	40,700
Healthways	429	10,000	74,000	150,000
Prucare	0	20,487	0	40,268
Elderplan	3,525	5,200	3,525	5,200
Maxicare	2,500	0	6,000	0
Metro	3,203	3,686	0	3,686
Kaiser	809	1,200	29,005	38,600
Other	N/A	6,981	N/A	38,568
Total	795,988	1,119,450	1,152,742	1,864,230

Sources: Crain's New York Business, August 24, 1987, and Crain's New York Business, August 27, 1990.

by the other firms. The first major membership source targeted by HMOs was the New York City municipal workers (approximately 400,000), but after an estimated expenditure of $50 million for marketing, less than 2 percent enrolled in HMOs and the vast majority of those opted either for HIP or Blue Cross. Within three years, having undergone little growth, Maxicare was forced to end its arrangement with the hospitals and withdrew completely from New York.

Alternative delivery systems have had only a minor impact on the hospital business. Because of the nature of the reimbursement system in the state, hospitals do not gain from offering HMOs a price discount, and given the high level of occupancy at New York City hospitals there is little need for increased admissions. Therefore HMOs have not been able to generate substantial discounts from New York hospitals—which may be a factor in their relatively slow growth there. The hospitals that have made arrangements with HMOs tend to be located in the outer boroughs and are those utilized by family practitioners. HMOs have attempted to utilize large group practices that operate primarily in the outer boroughs; only a minority of New York City physicians have arrangements with HMOs and therefore it appears that physicians who join one HMO panel, tend to join several.

The only ambulatory surgery sites (with the exception of surgery done in physicians' offices) are satellites of hospitals. Ambulatory diagnostic work and radiology, though, have grown rapidly due to the New York

State CON regulations that restrict the acquisition of high-tech equipment by hospitals. Many physician groups and private entrepreneurs have set up ambulatory facilities to meet the demand.

Health Workers

Physicians

In New York City a physician surplus coexists with a physician shortage. In 1989, fifty percent of the city's 23,000 physicians practiced in Manhattan, yet almost 50 percent of Manhattan's population lived in federally designated health manpower shortage areas. Thus there seems to be a concentration and centralization of physicians in primarily wealthy areas of the city and a shortage of physicians in nonwealthy areas.

The long, and growing, waiting lists of physicians seeking to gain admitting privileges at major New York City hospitals may be one sign of a physician surplus. An increasing number of surgeons willing to enter PPO-type arrangements (i.e., willing to accept lower fees in return for a greater volume of service) and the return of physician home visits in some outer-borough communities may be other signs of an oversupply of physicians in the metropolitan area.

At the same time, it has not been possible to get physicians to set up practices in low-income areas of the city, which remain medically underserved. In 1989, approximately 15 percent of the physicians in New York City billed Medicaid for services. An even lower percentage of dentists participated in the program. Analysis reveals that much of the physician billing is done from OPDs and clinics rather than from private practice sites. The current Medicaid payment for an office visit in New York is $11, but it has been estimated that the average cost per visit to a primary care physician in New York City is closer to $47. The state has been resistent to raising Medicaid fees for physicians for several reasons largely having to do with the increased cost and the limited return from such additional reimbursement. It would be politically difficult to give more money to physicians for care of the poor, particularly in an era of cutbacks of services. Moreover, raising the fees would only marginally induce new physicians to join the program, and the amount of money that it would take to make Medicaid fees competitive with private fees would be far greater than the state could afford. Finally, there is a widespread perception that the Medicaid program is abused by both providers and clients. Raising the fees without having a mechanism to control utilization of the program would increase demand far faster than supply could meet it, and in any event, the cost would be substantially more than would be anticipated.

New York State started a number of programs during the 1960s and 1970s to subsidize medical school tuition for state residents in return for a commitment to practice in underserved areas. Many of the beneficiaries of these programs have bought out (that is, paid off their loans plus interest), and many others have chosen not to serve in New York City. Moreover, the definition of "underserved area" that is utilized by the state allows doctors to work in hospitals and in any specialties, with the result that there is no necessary connection to the primary care needs of underserved populations. Since 1980 there have been attempts to establish programs to homestead physicians in the city. Physicians would be provided with office space and administrative support by a hospital and in some cases their malpractice premiums would be paid, in return for which they would accept indigent patients. A few such sites exist under the aegis of voluntary hospitals, but none have expanded in the past two years. The Health and Hospitals Corporation initiated such a program in 1985 which was terminated in 1988 because of its failure to attract participating physicians.

There appear to be few joint ventures between physicians and hospitals in New York City. Presbyterian Hospital has been the most significant exception to this rule, having set up a radiology group on the Upper East Side of Manhattan and a pediatrics group in an affluent section of the Bronx. Part of the explanation lies in the strictness of New York CON legislation, which implicitly outlawed joint ventures after the state determined that hospitals that had been denied CONs for equipment (e.g., CAT scanners) were making such arrangements with staff physicians (who were not covered by the regulation) and thus bypassing the state regulatory apparatus. As a result the state has monitored such joint ventures very closely.

It is more difficult to get a handle on other forms of entrepreneurialism. Physician groups have acquired high technology services that are often lacking in any but the major teaching hospitals, including radiology, radiotherapy, imaging, and lithotripsy. Hospitals report anecdotally, that physicians are using fewer ancillary services, suggesting that they may now be performing those tests and procedures in their offices. It is difficult to tease out information about the growth of entrepreneurialism from the statistics of health insurance carriers, which monitor hospital utilization far more intensively than they monitor office visits.

During the 1980s there was an increase in the number of full-time physicians working in hospitals. In New York City, their numbers were increasing even before the state placed restrictions on hospital house staff hours. Most New York City hospitals responded to the state regulations by hiring full-time staff rather than forcing attending physicians to provide more service to the hospitals. The director of the New York County

Medical Society reported that he had received no complaints from members of the society about the regulations and surmised that attending physicians have been almost totally isolated from the changes. Many hospitals have found it easy to hire full-time physicians (particularly member hospitals of the Health and Hospitals Corporation), which may be another indication of a physician surplus or, alternatively, simply of the difficulties of starting a private practice.

The only noticeable trend in physician supply has been a decline in the number of physicians in the outer boroughs (largely due to physicians retiring and not being replaced) and an increase in the number of physicians in Manhattan. The number of physicians in the surrounding metropolitan area seems to be growing, but this growth does not seem to be at the expense of doctors in New York City.

Nurses

In the latter part of the 1980s, New York, like other large cities, experienced a major nursing shortage, most acute at the hospitals belonging to the Health and Hospitals Corporation but severe at other hospitals as well. Most hospitals took to importing nurses from foreign countries (the West Indies, Ireland, and Canada were the sources of choice) and engaged in more extensive nurse recruiting. In 1989 the governor allowed for increased reimbursement to help hospitals pay higher nursing salaries, and union contracts pushed entry level salaries well above the $30,000 range for newly licensed nurses. Many hospitals closed beds and units because they lacked the staff to operate the beds, creating an occupancy crisis (the same number of patients and fewer beds). Other strategies for dealing with the nursing shortage have included upskilling of licensed practical nurses (LPNs), using more LPNs in place of registered nurses (RNs), and creating high schools of the health sciences to interest more young people in nursing and health careers in general.

Other Health Workers

New York City has experienced shortages in a variety of health worker categories. Hospital-based therapists of all kinds have been in short supply, as have other hospital-based workers, particularly those whose jobs exposed them to blood (presumably because of fear of contracting AIDS), as well as carpenters, plumbers, and other skilled maintenance workers who can find better pay outside the hospital. A 1987 study by the New York State Department of Health found either shortages or potential shortages in most health occupations in New York City and concluded that unless serious measures were taken to improve recruitment into the field, the shortages would worsen. The public hospital system because of its low wages, experienced more severe shortages than the voluntary system. Hospitals in general have fared better than nursing homes, which have fared better than home care agencies.

Medical Education

There were no changes in the number or size of New York City medical schools over the course of the study. Consideration was given to opening a new public medical school in Queens, but budgetary problems put this proposal on a back burner. Residency programs in major teaching hospitals continued to do well in attracting graduating medical students to fill their slots, but there is anecdotal information that New York City is becoming a less desirable place for house staff.

In the interest of cost control, the State Department of Health has attempted to cut back the amount of graduate medical education that is being provided through residency programs in New York hospitals. The argument is, first, that New York is bearing the costs and burdens of training physicians who will not practice in the state, and, second, that the more doctors trained, the greater the costs of medical care. Hence, the state has discussed but thus far not instituted regulations that would limit the number of residents that teaching hospitals may have. One proposal would establish teaching consortia based around area medical schools; each consortium would be allotted a finite number of residents to distribute to all of the hospitals in its geographic area. The objective of the plan would be the elimination of over 2,000 of 16,000 resident positions. However, the reaction to this and other proposals of similar intent has been negative and has evoked strong resistance from the hospitals and the medical schools.

The major development in medical education in New York during the decade was the battle between the State Board of Regents and the State Department of Health over whether graduates from certain foreign medical schools, principally from the Caribbean, should be eligible for licensure. The State Board of Regents is responsible for licensing health care professionals. In response to severe shortages of physicians in both inner city and rural areas of the state, the regents permitted students of off-shore medical schools to obtain medical externships in New York hospitals and recognized their medical degrees as qualifying for a New York State license. They reasoned that if the supply of doctors expanded sufficiently, economic circumstances would eventually force physicians to move into less desirable areas. At the same time, the State Department of Health was feeling the impact of these decisions through higher reimbursements paid to hospitals and greater medical care costs throughout the state. In a battle with the regents on the issue of quality of education obtained by the foreign medical graduates (FMGs), the Health Department finally persuaded the regents to disaccredit some of the foreign medical schools. It is interesting that, reminiscent of Flexnerian times, the general decline in applications to U.S. medical schools probably spelled the demise of these marginal schools just as surely as the proscriptions by New York State.

Indigent Care

The most recent data on the number of uninsured in New York City come from special analyses of Current Population Survey (CPS) data. Of the population under sixty-five, 18. 9 percent (1.3 million) were uninsured in 1985 and 15.5 percent (1.1 million) received Medicaid. Since then Medicaid enrollment and the number of uninsured have risen significantly. In 1990 there were an estimated 1.5 million uninsured and 1.35 million Medicaid recipients. Because the CPS is a household survey, the data probably undercount the uninsured, particularly those who are homeless. The majority of the uninsured in New York end up in HHC institutions either through the direct shifting of patients by voluntary hospitals, particularly those that are physically connected or proximate to public facilities (consider New York University Hospital and Bellevue for example; in 1989 NYU had 3.4 percent Medicaid in-patients, Bellevue 57.7 percent), or through policies that make it difficult for Medicaid enrollees or uninsured individuals to utilize the private hospitals (admission only by a private physician, payment in advance, etc.).

As the costs of outpatient care have risen, many voluntary hospitals have restricted access to their OPDs and clinics. Such restrictions have served to push even more people into HHC hospital clinics. It seems likely that this trend will continue unless the state increases its all-inclusive Medicaid rate (frozen since 1981) for OPD and ER visits. In 1989, two of the largest medical centers in Manhattan (Mount Sinai and Presbyterian) announced the closure of their outpatient pharmacies due to high cost.

The threshold for Medicaid eligibility in New York has remained relatively high, although it has fallen since the program was inaugurated in 1966. In 1989, the Medicaid ceiling for a family of four in New York was $7,400, whereas the federal poverty limit for a family of four was $11,000. It was not until 1988 that New York expanded the eligibility level for pregnant women to include those up to 185 percent of the poverty level in compliance with federal Omnibus Budget Reconciliation Act (OBRA) and Supplementary Omnibus Budget Reconciliation Act (SOBRA) regulations because of a lengthy fight between pro- and anti-choice legislators over the issue of coverage for abortions. In New York City (which pays 25 percent of the total Medicaid costs for its residents), the number of people enrolled in the program has grown from 1.1 to 1.3 million since 1980. The issue of shifting most of the burden of Medicaid (starting with long-term care) to the state government has been under discussion between the state and the counties for many years. The process has been slowed by policy disagreements as well as by an increasingly unfavorable budgetary situation within the state.

Since the start of the decade, the hospital reimbursement system in New York State has included a bad debt and charity care pool as a means of helping hospitals pay for the costs of the indigent. Financed by a tax on hospital revenues, which is redistributed according to the level of indigent care, the pool serves to funnel money from more profitable upstate hospitals to hospitals in New York City. Uncompensated services are fully reimbursed only for a few financially distressed hospitals in the state. Only a small portion of the fund is distributed to the public hospitals as a means of forcing them to maintain their level of commitment (that is, to keep the city from withdrawing money from the hospitals, given the availability of alternative funds). Some $600 million was redistributed in 1988 through the bad debt and charity care pool, almost 90 percent of it to New York City institutions. The pool does not reimburse for services provided in facilities other than hospitals (community health centers, primary care clinics, etc.), nor does it reimburse for physician services in any setting.

The growth in the number of the uninsured has had a profound impact on the organization of services in New York City. In the period just before the implementation of Medicare and Medicaid, many health policy analysts entertained the possibility of dismantling the public hospital system in New York because, with the introduction of these entitlement programs, it would no longer serve any useful purpose. It has become clear, in the years since, that the need for public hospitals remains as great or greater than before the introduction of federal financing for the poor and the elderly. The volume of uninsured patients in New York has grown so rapidly that they can no longer be accommodated solely within the public hospital system. As the dimensions of poverty have extended geographically, hospitals outside the public system have also become responsible for the care of indigent patients, with an increasingly dire impact on their financial stability. Nowhere is this situation more evident than at Presbyterian Hospital in northern Manhattan. Once the enclave of the upper and upper middle classes in northern Manhattan and New Jersey, the hospital has largely become the province of indigent Hispanic residents of Washington Heights, Inwood, and nearby neighborhoods in the Bronx. With no public hospitals in the vicinity to receive indigent patients, Presbyterian has gone from one of the wealthiest hospitals in the United States to one that lost $33 million in operating costs in 1989. The deluge of uninsured patients has served to keep paying patients away from the facility (both because beds are scarce and because the wealthy have other options in more attractive locations), which further worsens the financial situation of the hospital.

Emergency rooms in New York City have also borne the burden of the rising uninsured population. In many hospitals with large emergency rooms, patients without private physicians are increasingly being admitted to the hospital through the ER. As a result, beds cannot be reserved in advance even for private patients, who must also wait in the queue at the emergency room.

Only anecdotal evidence is available by which to assess the state of access to health services in New York City. It seems clear that access decreased significantly over the past decade. Not only were the number of hospital beds cut, but reductions in the number of beds that are actually staffed and operated even further diminished the capacity of the system to respond to need. We know that the number of uninsured in New York rose, and we know that poverty grew worse. We know that the quality of health insurance decreased as well. Some say that access is no worse today than it was ten years ago and that it is just more visible—chiefly because of the growth in homelessness. Yet, occupancy rates are higher for a smaller number of beds, and emergency rooms have never been as backlogged.

To the extent that the problem of the uninsured has been addressed at all, it has been viewed as a state or national problem. Given the large commitment of resources that New York City gives to health services for the poor—both hospital and non-hospital services—there is a feeling within city government that any further provision of service must be financed by either the state or federal government. The New York State Department of Health floated a proposal entitled UNY*Care that would create a state health insurance program with a single payer for services and universal coverage. The proposal was introduced in the spring of 1989 and is not currently a major contender in the health policy debate, but it does indicate the state's sense of responsibility for assuring adequate health services to its residents. In effect, the state is saying that access to health services is largely a New York City issue that the city cannot address; that it is really a federal responsibility that the federal government will not address, and so, by default, the state must deal with it.

In a more prosperous period, it is possible that UNY*Care or a similar proposal would get a better hearing, but the fiscal condition of the state in 1990 (with its multibillion dollar, and growing, deficit) precludes any major financing initiative. Even if cost were not an issue, the proposal would have a difficult time politically because it makes the state the single payer of services. Both hospitals and physicians would vigorously fight against the state's assumption of this role. Given the struggle of the hospitals to get out from under the thumb of the state as the sole payer (by eliminating the Medicare waiver), it is doubtful that they would revert to a similar position. It is also doubtful that physicians would cede to the state control over their potential incomes.

Public Health Issues

New York City remains at the epicenter of AIDS after a decade of devastation by the disease. Perhaps the most significant development has been the shift in the epidemic from a largely white, middle-class, insured, gay population to a minority, underclass, uninsured drug-using population. This shift has altered both the geography of the disease and the mechanisms through which treatment is financed. By 1990, the number of cases of AIDS that had been diagnosed in New York City was 29,443, and the number of deaths was 16,801 (57.0 percent).

Hospitals in New York have been reporting a large increase in the number of patients who are in need of treatment for mental illnesses. There is a widespread perception that many if not most homeless people were mentally ill before they became homeless or quickly became mentally ill after losing their homes.

Infectious diseases, particularly measles and tuberculosis (TB) have been on the upsurge since 1985. Some association exists between TB and AIDS, but the exact relation remains unclear.

Estimates that over 250,000 New Yorkers are drug abusers are frequently heard, but the validity of the number is unclear. There has been an increase in the abuse of certain drugs, particularly crack. Usage of other drugs, such as powdered cocaine, seems to have fallen off.

Sexually transmitted diseases are on the increase in New York City, as they have been around the country. In December 1989, the city health department reinstituted mandatory testing of newborns for syphilis due to the rising frequency of new cases. The procedure had been discontinued because of low cost-effectiveness in the mid-1970s.

Infant mortality rates were on the increase in the late 1980s, particularly in minority communities. After a long period of decline, the rates leveled off and then started their recent upsurge. Along with infant mortality rates, other indicators of worsening health status, including the number of births with late or no prenatal care and the frequency of low-birth-weight babies, are also on the rise. As with most of the conditions that have been described, the deterioration in health status has hit minority and poor communities the hardest.

Public health budgets in New York City sank to a low in the period immediately after 1975 as a consequence of the city's fiscal crisis. This situation was exacerbated by the introduction of federal block grants, a new strategy for paying for public health services that effectively reduced the amount of grant funding. Since the period of the fiscal crisis, the city health department has given up most of its direct service responsibilities and has eliminated most child health, well-baby, and dental clinics. It remains responsible for health protection and health promotion activities.

There has been some movement to integrate public health functions with the corpus of the medical care delivery system. Specifically, New York City began a program in 1986 that attempted to place well-child clinics in public hospital outpatient departments. Earlier, expanded school health functions were given to specially trained health resource coordinators who worked for the health department but who were based in junior and senior high schools. That program was defunded in 1990.

Homelessness increased greatly over the period of the study. The impact of the problem on the health system is reflected in many ways. Through their encounters with staff, patients, and visitors in hospitals, homeless patients suffering from infectious and contagious diseases are spreading these pathologies to an otherwise unexposed population; homeless mothers are giving birth to crack-addicted and AIDS-infected babies. Children raised for long periods of time in homeless environments present special emotional and psychological problems. The estimates for 1990 of 14,000 homeless families in New York City may be on the low side. These estimates do not count persons who live with relatives or friends in crowded, small apartments and who may be only a step away from true homelessness.

Conclusions

The health system of New York City in the early 1990s does not look dramatically, different from that of 1980. Institutionally and organizationally it has changed only slightly. Perhaps the biggest changes are related to the imperative of dealing with problems such as AIDS that were nonexistent in 1980 and with others that have assumed vastly greater dimensions since then—drug abuse, homelessness, the uninsured.

The major national events had, in the aggregate, little impact on the New York City health system. The state had a waiver from the PPS system until 1986, and so DRGs for Medicare patients were irrelevant. The state retained its health planning program and certificate of need regulations after the federal government defunded the program nationally. HMOs and PPOs made little headway in New York City, and fee-for-service medicine provided by solo practitioners retained its hegemony.

Academic health centers continued to dominate health care delivery in New York City, and the rebuilding and modernization of the major academic health centers over the decade further entrenched the dominant tertiary care orientation. Much was said about primary care over the decade, but little was done about it.

The principal determinant of change within the health system appears to be the combination of the state health reimbursement policy and local, institutional factors. State health reimbursement policy is crucial in New York City because the state utilizes an all-payer system (which now excludes Medicare). Thus any change in reimbursement policy has a dramatic impact on the entire hospital system or other segment of the health delivery system. Further, inasmuch as the state controls access to capital and new technology (through the CON program), institutional health care delivery is in thrall to state policy.

Because the health institutions in New York City are so large, and most have a long history, change does not come easily. Resistance to change is abetted by a substantial access to philanthropy, by the presence of a large number of medical schools, and by the high cost of change. The entrenched system is of course influenced by external factors and events, but it is fair to say that none of those that were noted during the 1980s has had profound consequences thus far. We have utilized a relatively narrow window as an observation point, and it is possible that a decade from now things will be viewed differently. At present, though, local and institutional factors are far greater determinants of change than are federal or other external events.

Bibliography

Altman, S., Garfink, C., *The Impact of the Federal Prospective Payment System on New York Hospitals* (Waltham, MA: Bigel Institute for Health Policy, 1989).

American Hospital Association, *Guide to the Health Care Field* (Chicago: American Hospital Association, 1980–1990).

Beauchamp, D., Rouse, R., "Universal New York Health Care," *The New England Journal of Medicine* 323 (September 6, 1990): 640–644.

Brecher, C., *The City of New York's* 1988 Preliminary Budget (New York: Citizens Budget Commission, 1987).

Brecher, C., Horton, R., *Setting Municipal Priorities* 1980 (Montclair, NJ: Allanheld Osmun, 1979).

_____ . *Setting Municipal Priorities* 1982 (New York: Russell Sage Foundation, 1981).

_____ . *Setting Municipal Priorities* 1984 (New York: New York University Press, 1983).

Center on Budget and Policy Priorities, *Holes in the Safety Nets: Poverty Programs and Policies in the States* (Washington, D.C.: Center on Budget and Policy Priorities, 1988).

Citizens Budget Commission, *Summary of New York City and New York State Finances: Fiscal Year* 1990–91 (New York: Citizens Budget Commission, 1990).

Dine, D., "Market Focus: New York," *Modern Healthcare* 19 (February 17, 1989): 40–46.

Community Service Society of New York, *Building Primary Health Care in New York Low-Income Communities* (New York: Community Service Society of New York, 1990).

Greater New York Hospital Association, *Statistics 89* (New York: Greater New York Hospital Association, 1989).

Health Systems Agency of New York City, *The Health Labor Force in New York City in the Year 2000* (New York: Health Systems Agency of New York, 1990).

———. *HIV/AIDS Data Book* (New York: Health Systems Agency of New York, 1990).

———. *AIDS Task Force Report* (New York: Health Systems Agency of New York, 1989).

———. *Profiles of New York City Hospitals: 1988–1989* (New York: Health Systems Agency of New York, 1990).

HMOs in New York City, *Crain's New York Business*, August, 1987, 1990.

New York City Department of Health, *Health of the City* (New York: Department of Health, 1989) .

New York City Health and Hospitals Corporation, *Assessment of Demographic Projections* (New York: Health and Hospitals Corporation, 1990).

———. *HMO Growth and Its Implications for New York City* (New York: Health and Hospitals Corporation, 1990).

———. *HHC: An Overview* (New York: Health and Hospitals Corporation, 1990).

———. *Caring for the Medically Uninsured* (New York: Health and Hospitals Corporation, 1989).

———. *New York City's Medically Uninsured: Summary Data* (New York: Health and Hospitals Corporation, 1988).

———. *The Crisis: Overcrowding in New York City Public Hospitals* (New York: Health and Hospitals Corporation, 1988).

———. *Key Background Information* (New York: Health and Hospitals Corporation, 1987).

New York State Department of Health, *Universal New York Health Care* (New York: Department of Health, 1989).

———. Bureau of Health Facility Planning, *Occupancy Quarterly Report* (New York: Department of Health, 1987–1989).

United Hospital Fund of New York, *Health and Health Care in New York City* (New York: United Hospital Fund, 1980–1990).

———. *Health Care Annual* (New York: United Hospital Fund, 1980–1990).

———. *Health Facilities in Southern New York* (New York: United Hospital Fund, 1975–1990).

———. *New York City's Hospital Utilization Crisis: A Background Paper* (New York: United Hospital Fund, 1987).

———. *Inpatient Hospital Use in New York* (New York: United Hospital Fund, 1985–1987).

———. *Ambulatory Care in New York* (New York: United Hospital Fund, 1984).

3

Chicago Health Care: Private Growth Amidst Public Stagnation

J. Warren Salmon

Health care trends in metropolitan Chicago during the 1980s reflect the changes witnessed in the American health care delivery system during the same period. The metropolitan region experienced a huge increase in the numbers of physicians, nurses, pharmacists, dentists, administrative staff, and other health workers; substantial growth in the size and influence of academic medical centers and teaching hospitals, for which Chicago is quite famous; a loss of fifteen community hospitals in the city alone; an unanticipated decline in hospital utilization; wide diversification of health care facilities beyond inpatient services and the accompanying growth in ambulatory services; the arrival of a whole set of new players (from new organizational forms to out-of-state health care corporations and large insurance companies); and a continued rise in governmental outlays for health care despite cost containment policies.

In the early 1990s the configuration of the local system reveals the prior decade's trends toward amalgamation and diversification beyond the hospital trends that are encountering even greater competitive and financial constraints today. This reshaping was surely not easy for locally based traditional health care providers and is by no means completed.

On the demand side, cost-containment forces now dictate the nature and terms of health care delivery. A changing demographic and epidemiologic profile for the city, county, and metropolitan region will have significant future impacts. For example, access to quality care remains a critical problem for one third of the Chicago population. It is estimated that 1.6 million people in Chicago—more than half of the total population—either are completely uninsured, have inadequate health insurance coverage, or are Medicaid recipients. The explosion in the ranks of the medically indigent occurred at the same time that the local public health care sector has become overburdened and underfunded. A new competitive bidding mechanism by the state Medicaid program—the Illinois Competitive Access and Reimbursement Equity, or ICARE program—was instituted in 1985 for hospital reimbursement; the Illinois Department of Public Aid now pays far less than costs to hospitals and delays payments to all providers by nearly ninety days. Private providers are thus discouraged from treating even Medicaid recipients, let alone "unsponsored" patients.

In the private insurance sector, Blue Cross/Blue Shield of Illinois continues to lose market share in the metropolitan region as employers self-insure and the share of commercial insurance companies has grown. HMOs, PPOs, and other forms of managed care are now prevalent and influential, although they have decreased in number as market shares have led to consolidations among fewer, stronger firms. Business groups are pressuring against cost-shifting within hospitals at the same time that federal funding cutbacks and the Medicare prospective payment system are limiting past options within the shrinking pool of providers.

The major dilemma for Chicago, as well as for the metropolitan region, is how to extend access to the growing number of medically indigent in a competitive marketplace driven by bottom-line objectives. These market forces are coupled with significant stagnation among the city, county, and state public providers and programs.

Demographics and Economics

Although America's population grew by about 10 percent during the 1980s, that of Illinois grew only by 2 percent, and the state held its position as the sixth largest state in the Union. In 1990 it was estimated that the state had 11,712,000 residents, of whom over 1.7 million were black, 755,000 were Hispanic, and more than 262,000 were other minorities.

The city of Chicago has not grown at all in population since 1970. The 2,783,726 Chicago residents in 1990 represented a decline of 7. 4 percent from the previous decade. Cook County had 5,105,067 residents in 1990, making it the second largest county in the nation. The Chicago standard metropolitan statistical area (SMSA) which comprises Cook, Kane, Lake, McHenry, and Will counties, accounts for the huge growth of the region to over 7 million people today.

The population of Chicago is projected to decline over the next twenty years, and is likely to undergo a marked, continuing shift in its racial/ethnic composition. This shift is expected to affect the age structure and socioeconomic makeup of the city. The 1990 census found a population approximately 42 percent black (skewed to the younger age groups), less than 36 percent white (skewed to the aged), and 18 percent Hispanic (skewed to the young also). Asians and other minorities made up around 4 percent of the 1990 census figures; Asians are the fastest growing group in Chicago. The younger distribution of the non-white population is reflected in Chicago's public school programs, which are over 60 percent black and 24 percent Hispanic. Illegal immigrants from Latin America (and Poland and Ireland, for that matter) have also flocked to the city, affecting ethnic composition.

As a city, Chicago's history is marked by both a strong neighborhood tradition (often segregated) and an uneven economic development among communities. Thus, changes in demographics are combined with epidemiologic factors (such as the greater prevalence of certain disease entities and higher birth/fertility rates among blacks and Hispanics) have produced varying health status profiles for different communities.

The aging of the city's white population, on the one hand, and the phenomenal growth in the number of the young among minorities, on the other, project an increasingly bimodal age distribution, with younger members predominating. The number of elderly persons in Cook County alone increased 12 percent during the 1980s, adding nearly 70,000 over-sixty-five years of age residents to the 562,000 in 1980. In 1985, more than $2 billion in Medicare funds poured into Chicago, accounting for 39 percent of gross patient revenues. As the federal government adopts ever more stringent reimbursement policies, hospital care for the aged becomes highly problematic.

Welfare rolls in Illinois remained relatively stable over the decade; however, this fact in no way means that there are fewer poor people. In fact, quite the opposite is true. State cuts over the decade were most acute for the Aid to Families with Dependent Children (AFDC) program; its allotments for families were frozen for an eight-year period, with the 1989 state budget providing a very small increment in monthly payments. Some cuts in Medicaid in the early part of the decade limited numbers of eligible persons, particularly for the categories of Aid to the Medically Indigent and General Assistance. Recent federal mandates liberalizing eligibility requirements for pregnant women may permit more Illinois women and children to enroll in the program statewide. In September 1989, there were approximately 641,000 recipients of public aid in the metro area, whereas only two years prior there were over 671,000 as calculated by the Metropolitan Chicago Healthcare Council. Since the economic recession squarely hit the Midwest in late 1990, welfare rolls in Illinois began to feel pressures to increase, though the same phenomena held true that greater numbers of poor and near poor people still do not receive state assistance.

The implications of these demographic developments are vital for public health policy. In and of themselves, they should strengthen arguments for mounting primary care and preventive strategies as means to contain future health care costs and to ease the growing burden on providers for end-stage interventions.

The economy of Illinois (the fifth largest state economy in the nation) appears much better in the early 1990s than at any time over the last decade, though no "boom" is expected. In 1990, the total gross state product was approximately $261.4 billion, or 5 percent of the GNP. Although per capita income for the nation was near $18,000, Chicago's was only $13,000. Unemployment was at a record ten-year low in Illinois (5.5 percent in September 1989); the rate for the metro area was 5.3 percent. Jobs were increasing steadily (5.2 million in 1989) due to a surge in the service sector (28 percent of all jobs). Manufacturing has been declining since the service sector began to exceed the manufacturing sector in number of jobs in the early 1980s. City job growth for 1986-1989 was only 5 percent (compared to the metro area's growth of 12.8 percent and suburban DuPage County's growth of 30.7 percent), though employment in the city is now at its highest level since 1981. However, the service sector's growth continues to be a long-term weak spot in the Illinois economy relative to national growth rates. The state is also reported by the U.S. Census Bureau to lag in health care growth. Many new jobs are part-time or relatively low paying and usually do not include health insurance as a fringe benefit. With the recent economic recession of 1990-1992 unemployment began to zoom, changing the overall favorable trend of the past decade. Across the 1980s, as well as predictably into the 1990s, employment, even when favorable, does little to ameliorate the uncompensated care problem of metro Chicago health providers. Thus, these overall favorable employment trends may do little to ameliorate the uncompensated-care problem of the metro Chicago health providers.

Over the decade of the 1980s, the development-underdevelopment tension within Chicago's economy was exacerbated. Civic pride (and developer greed) vis-à-vis the downtown Loop building boom overshadowed strategies to minimize the significant declines among inner-city communities, including the demise of city manufacturing and small commercial businesses. Most of the growth in city jobs mentioned previously was for jobs in the downtown Super Loop area. The gentrification of certain neighborhoods has saved some health providers from financial ruin, whereas its obverse has taken its toll among community hospitals and clinics that are unable to attract paying patients to seek treatment in their squalid surroundings. Gentrification also exacerbated the housing crisis among lower-income Chicagoans, adding to homelessness and its attending social pathologies. Public housing in Chicago remains a disaster, and virtually no help is being offered to the growing numbers of homeless people. In addition, the conversion of buildings formerly used for manufacturing into lofts and condominiums for middle-class professionals represents a further erosion of the economic base.

The Health Care Structure and Establishment

Within the Chicago area are the national headquarters for the American Medical Association, the American Dental Association, the American College of Surgeons, the American College of Health Care Executives, the American Hospital Association, the Joint Commission on Accreditation of Healthcare Organizations, the Blue Cross/Blue Shield Association, and over one hundred other national health professional groups. However, their general interface with and influence upon metropolitan providers and policymakers (except in the areas of medical research and product development) is quite scanty.

The wealth of medical research performed in the Chicago area has encouraged the growth of manufacturing in science-based industries. Several major corporate suppliers (e.g., Pfizer, Searle, Abbott Laboratories, Baxter, Borg-Warner, FMC Chicago, and Whitman Industries) add to the health care industry by being headquartered in the region.

The presence of academic teaching and research institutions also has had a major influence upon the regional health care system. However, no Chicago hospitals are usually listed in surveys of the top ten health care institutions in the nation. Unlike their peers in New York City, upper-class Chicagoans often travel to medical centers of excellence elsewhere for specialty care. Nevertheless, medical research is carried out in eighty-one universities, hospitals, laboratories, and foundations in the city, with other suburban facilities adding to this concentration.

Seven medical schools are located in the metropolitan area: the University of Chicago, Northwestern, Rush, University of Illinois, Chicago Osteopathic, Loyola (in suburban Cook County), and the University of Health Sciences–Chicago Medical School (in Lake County). Along with the five Chicago-based academic medical centers, there are eight other major teaching hospitals in the city proper. Significant variations are found in the type of academic affiliation that exists between each medical school and its different teaching hospitals. Only within the past several years have a few of the medical schools initiated more advanced multi-institutional systems for administrative and clinical purposes. Such arrangements seem to be more prevalent in other areas across the nation.

Corporatization Trends

Among the teaching institutions, changes in ownership have recently occurred within the larger metropolitan area. A reason for this emergent pattern is that new powers can be brought together to secure their market shares among the well-insured middle class, particularly in the suburbs. During the period 1988-1990, multi-institutional relationships spurted. Whereas religious-sponsored institutions amalgamated earlier in the decade, we now see regionalization efforts led by academic medical centers and their affiliated hospitals. Rush-Presbyterian–St. Luke's Medical Center merged with Copley Memorial Hospital in west suburban Aurora in 1988, following a merger with Skokie Valley Community Hospital (now Rush–North Shore) in 1987. The University of Chicago Hospital (UC) combined with Louis A. Weiss Memorial Hospital in the Uptown community subsequent to the aborted UC merger with Michael Reese Hospital on the South Side. Northwestern Memorial Hospital created the largest network, composed of its medical school teaching affiliates: Children's Memorial Medical Center, Chicago; the Rehabilitation Institute of Chicago; Highland Park Hospital; and Evanston Hospital Corporation, which operates Evanston Hospital as well as Glenbrook Hospital in Glenview. This Northwestern McGaw group, which will have a combined annual revenue of about $719 million in 1990, is seeking a total of ten to twelve hospitals for its network. An amalgamation on a smaller scale in 1990 united two Catholic groups on the Northwest Side and suburbs: The new entity, the Chicago Catholic Healthcare System, Inc., is composed of a hospital from the Resurrection Health Care Corporation and one from the Alexian Brothers of Illinois, Inc.

The most publicized, though never implemented, organizational arrangement was the proposed affiliation of the University of Illinois College of Medicine with Michael Reese Hospital and Medical Center. Because the state legislature refused to allow the university to lease its own facility to the government of Cook County on a long-term basis and to make Reese its primary affiliate, the relationship was reduced to an academic tie-in. Three years later, the Michael Reese board sold out to the for-profit Humana Corporation, based in Louisville, Kentucky, which intends to extend its Humana-Reese HMO network across the metropolitan area.

The College of Osteopathic Medicine operates a suburban medical center, Olympia Fields, in addition to its South Side Chicago hospital. Its diversification plans entail the establishment of a new B.S. degree pharmacy school and other allied health training programs in DuPage County. Earlier, each of the allopathic medical schools had spun off its hospital as a separate corporation; in contrast, the University of Illinois Medical School and hospital continue to be governed by the same board of trustees.

In terms of political power, Chicago's teaching institutions have been largely unsuccessful in preventing the Illinois Medicaid program from shifting a major portion of inpatient care to lower-cost hospitals under the ICARE program and from underpaying for the care that they retained. The teaching hospitals are not notable for their political clout in the state legislature, as evidenced by their failure to obtain funding for the Chicago trauma care system.

Over the last decade, the multi-institutional health care chain became a regional phenomenon, especially among the church-sponsored institutions. The largest provider of health care in the area continues to be the Evangelical Health System (EHS), which now encompasses six hospitals and other diversified services. EHS is sponsored by the United Church of Christ. Lutheran General Health System had been the second largest not-for-profit health corporation, but with the closing of Lutheran General–Lincoln Park, it has been overtaken by the Northwestern and Rush systems. For most of the decade the Adventist Health System, based in Arlington, Texas, operated a few religiously affiliated hospitals in the area. In May 1989, these hospitals were incorporated within the Hinsdale Health System, a newly formed regional affiliate of Adventist. Several Catholic systems, for example, the Daughters of Charity, maintain groups of hospitals throughout the geographic region. As in other jurisdictions, there were several abortive attempts at system consolidation and start-up. These included Lutheran General System–EHS; the University of Chicago–Michael Reese; the University of Illinois–Michael Reese; and Grant–Lutheran General–Lincoln Park, to name but a few.

In 1987 the Catholic Health Alliance for Metropolitan Chicago was formed for the purpose of organizing joint ventures and establishing a PPO among the area's twenty-three (now twenty-one) Catholic hospitals. (Sixteen different religious orders own and manage these institutions.) This Catholic federation has been slow to galvanize the hospitals' chief executive officers, the orders, and their systems to act. St. Anne's Hospital is now closed, and several of the remaining Catholic hospitals are at risk for closure. Still, the hospitals in the federation control almost 4,000 beds, or nearly a quarter of the city's total acute-care capacity, and provide substantial uncompensated care for Chicagoans. As with the Evangelical and Lutheran General systems, Catholic orders seem to honor their historical commitments by maintaining money-losing operations in medically underserved Chicago communities. Given their inner-city commitment (location might be a better descriptor), one might think that Catholic and other religiously oriented private institutions should exert greater pressure for increased public financing of care for the Medicaid and indigent populations.

Had the Chicago Archdiocese not run into a financial catastrophe by 1990, it may have been able to provide the necessary leadership for the Catholic hospitals to lobby for greater state, and perhaps county, support of private sector strategies for indigent care. However, it has never been a major player in health care in Chicago and has not attempted to unify health policy among Catholic hospitals, though the Catholic Charities has been relatively important as a leader and advocate for social service agencies. The growing Hispanic and Southeast Asian communities face critical problems with access to health and human services and often prefer Catholic community hospitals and agencies. However, Catholic politics in Chicago (with its divisions among the individual orders that operate the hospitals), the financial gravity of parish schools, the closing of historical churches, and an eroding attendance at church services, all constrain any efforts to alter the maldistribution of health care.

Various motivations lie behind these overall changes in ownership and this organizational restructuring, but the major impetus for the systems is clearly financial: to broaden their geographic reach, establish feeder networks, expand their scope and control of services beyond the hospital, maximize investment, streamline management and minimize certain expenses, and, ultimately, wield greater market power. Such organizational patterns among these not-for-profit institutions often carry with them subtle reorientations of mission, which raise considerable concern among the public and professionals alike. Interestingly, religious leaders and congregations in Chicago are expressing concern that "their" hospitals are not doing more for the mounting needs within the inner city.

Proprietarization Trends

With respect to the role of for-profit ownership and management of health facilities and programs in Illinois, the state was, in the past, an attractive market to certain out-of-state hospital management firms, HMOs, nursing home chains, home health care companies, and even the nation's first for-profit hospice corporation. As in other areas nationally, fewer strategic bases are now being sought by for-profit chains in the middle-class suburbia surrounding Chicago, a retreat from the pattern earlier in the decade. However, the Humana takeover of Michael Reese Hospital represents a resurgence of the initial intrusion.

Several national for-profit health care systems operate in Illinois: Hospital Corporation of America (HCA), Humana, National Medical Enterprises (NME), Charter Medical, Forum Health Investors, and Universal Health Systems. Hospital ownership by these large corporate firms is not widespread, though contract management for hospitals has increased throughout the metropolitan region. The Federation of American Health Systems, the national trade association of the for-profit health care systems, noted that records of such contracts may be underreported.

With regard to the relation of the for-profit systems to academic medical centers, HCA signed a three-year management contract with the University of Illinois Eye and Ear Institute in 1987. Construction of a proposed 300-bed facility by Humana for the Chicago Medical School in Lake County was planned and later canceled. Some analysts felt that Humana exerted undue influence on the state health planning agency to upset local agency decisions not to build that hospital in the overbedded area of Lake County. Humana was also a failed suitor of St. Theresa Hospital in Waukegan, rejected as the result of a Vatican decision that prevailed upon another Catholic order to keep this financially plagued institution in the faith.

Among the more dramatic episodes in Chicago health care during the 1980s were the decline of the 652-bed Michael Reese Hospital and Medical Center from its historical stature and record of accomplishment through an abortive University of Chicago Hospital merger; the termination of Reese's participation in the city trauma network; a debacle when the University of Illinois College of Medicine attempted to make Reese its primary teaching hospital; and then the buy-out of Reese by Humana. Humana reportedly offered more money for the Michael Reese Health Plan alone than the amount ($90 million) involved in taking over the hospital. The acquisition of the Michael Reese Health Plan (the area's second largest HMO) has enabled Humana to move aggressively toward becoming the area leader. In the aftermath of the sought-after University of Chicago and University of Illinois bailouts, Reese's financial plight (the hospital reported a $17 million loss in 1989) was exacerbated by the flight of medical staff and traditional Jewish donors. With the Humana takeover, charitable support was withdrawn completely as some of the most prominent Chicago philanthropists were ironically wooed to archrival Rush. The Humana management has requested to keep the University of Illinois teaching affiliation through 1995, but deep concerns about Humana's intentions are prevalent among competing hospitals, as well as among the vulnerable South Side black and Hispanic communities that Reese had previously served. With its Medicaid proportion approaching 30 percent, Reese provided $19.5 million in uncompensated care in 1989. Several observers suspect that Humana's interest in the 240,000 enrollees of the health plan may lead it to concentrate exclusively on an HMO strategy and eventually sell off portions of the fifty-eight-acre Reese lakeside campus. The $29 million purchase price of the Reese Hospital represented a discount of 72 percent from the value of the property and equipment.

As for proprietary operations in the city itself, Universal Health Systems, Charter Medical, Humana, and Forum Health Investors each own one hospital; and HCA owns two. Two other proprietary hospitals are not affiliated with corporate chains. Except for the Universal facility and Lakeside Community Hospital, the for-profit institutions are psychiatric/substance abuse treatment centers. Thus, there are eight hospitals owned by for-profit organizations in Chicago. The immediate surrounding area has eight proprietary hospitals, including those belonging to HCA,

Humana, and Community Psychiatric Hospitals. As of 1991, there were twenty-two proprietaries in the state.

The Health Care Establishment

Beyond the power of individual institutional providers, several professional associations and societies exert considerable influence on public policy formulation. Something of a rivalry exists between the Illinois Hospital Association (IHA) and the Metropolitan Chicago Healthcare Council (MCHC), formerly the Chicago Hospital Council. Both have sizable staffs that work in the overall interest of their member institutions. Their activities include everything from lobbying and public relations to group purchasing and shared services.

A more powerful organization in the health policy arena, at least during the twelve years of former Governor James Thompson's administration, has been the Illinois State Medical Society (ISMS). (The governor's father, a radiologist at Bethany Hospital, was an officer of the ISMS.) Organized medicine's ability to block legislation and obtain administrative acquiescence to its positions is notorious. Major tort reform, an increase in the Medicaid physician reimbursement, and minimal government interference in the practice of medicine preoccupy its agenda for preserving its members' prerogatives. A past president attempted to muzzle, if not remove, the editor of the *Journal of the American Medical Association* (*JAMA*) for criticism of the house of medicine. The ISMS is reported to be sometimes underhanded in its politicking, along with being generally unrepresentative. Less than half of the practicing physicians in the state are members; the other physicians seem more dedicated to a variety of medical groups organized along ethnic lines. The latter have not been very vocal in espousing alternative viewpoints to those of the Illinois State Medical Society, which has been particularly effective in creating a public image, and convincing many state legislators, that it speaks for all physicians. The involvement of persons from academic medicine in the Chicago Medical Society (CMS), which has jurisdiction over Cook County, may account for the difference of its tone on certain policy issues. For example, a past president gained the endorsement of the CMS to the principle of access for all citizens to basic medical care. The participation of the CMS in the Chicago and Cook County Health Care Summit was praised by several health activists, and reform-minded physicians have become increasingly active in the CMS leadership.

All of these professional associations were given a role in the Health Care Summit, convened in 1989 by Governor Thompson, Cook County Board President George Dunne, and Mayor Richard Daley, to address public health care delivery in Cook County. This group was charged with the mission of suggesting a restructuring of the services rendered by the city, county, and state, the latter represented primarily by the University of Illinois Hospital and Clinics.

Political support for public health issues, Medicaid funding, and matters of public health care delivery in Chicago and Illinois remains embarrassingly scant compared to what occurs in other large industrial states and major cities. In the opinion of several observers, the general apathy may be partly due to the lack of an involved leadership from the business sector and partly to the preoccupation of grass-roots community and consumer constituencies with issues other than health care. Whereas the corporate sector mobilized around school reform in Chicago, there seems to be a persistent indifference to health matters—although a few concerned persons may be stimulating some positive response. The Midwest Business Group on Health has served primarily larger employers with educational programs mainly featuring ideas for containing employee health benefits. The organization does not participate in local conflicts with providers, although some of its counterparts around the nation have done so. A minor interest in health care has been shown by the Executive Service Corps, which has been involved in inner-city neighborhoods chiefly in the area of educational reform. The Civic Federation monitors taxation and spending by the county and city and has lately been more attuned to health issues. Chicago United, a civic organization representing minority businesses, has looked at health problems but has yet to become active in any projects. The Civic Committee of the Commercial Club—essentially made up of the major corporations in the city—has observed health issues from afar, mostly dreaming of a Houston-styled world-class medical center on the Westside for economic development purposes. The staff at the Chicago Association of Commerce and Industry, which represents smaller businesses, also dabble in health care issues, but so far they have done so without consequence. The state's small business lobby successfully blocked an IHA proposal for mandatory insurance to cover uncompensated charges for the state's 620,000 uninsured workers; Illinois labor unions naturally supported this legislation, but they appear to be more concerned with workers' compensation reform and employee health benefit cutbacks. A broad state-wide coalition of consumer and labor groups has formed around the campaign for Better Health Care, which has lobbied for a universal, single-payer state health insurance initiative.

Organized labor also has shown little concern for, and influence in, local health care politics beyond its representation of health workers. The main concern of a battered health force union has been job retention or, perhaps more accurately, membership retention. Relatively small numbers of the health care workers in the Chicago area have been organized by the Illinois Nurses Association; the American Federation of State, County and Municipal Employees; the Service Employees International Union; and the National Physicians Housestaff Association—the last only at Cook County Hospital. Over the decade, Chicago area hospitals mounted a concerted campaign to bust health worker unions and limit their advances; individually and collectively, these unions exert minimum influence in Chicago as compared to New York.

The lack of support from the business sector and organized labor for health care reform and the preoccupation of grass-roots community groups with nonhealth issues are noteworthy, especially considering the backwardness of the public health sector and the neglect of community health improvements by private health providers. Crucial leadership has not come forth from any of these camps, which has allowed public policy to stagnate under the control of uninformed and unconcerned politicians.

For a comprehensive understanding of the health care establishment, note should be taken of the overriding influence of the Illinois Department of Public Aid (IDPA) as a major payer (over $2 billion in 1990) and of the Illinois Department of Public Health (IDPH) as a regulator, convener, and sometimes "moral leader" on public policy issues. IDPA is generally thought of by certain providers, legal aid, and advocacy groups as an administrative remnant of the 1950s. Its Illinois Competitive Access and Reimbursement Equity (ICARE) program for purchasing hospital care for Medicaid recipients under competitive bidding exacerbated tensions between the public and private health sectors. Hospitals claim significant underpayment for care which resulted from IDPA cost-cutting even prior to the implementation of ICARE in 1985. The poor often have really only one option in obtaining care—public providers. Antagonisms have eased as small beginnings are made to expand Medicaid benefit levels and to make the bureaucracy more responsive. In 1989 hospitals were able to obtain disproportionate share funding for Medicaid in lieu of increasing ICARE rates. However, the new governor, Jim Edgar, has slowed provider payments to approximately a ninety-day cycle and has refused to budget sufficiently to keep the Medicaid program solvent.

The state-designated Illinois Health Care Cost Containment Council (IHCCCC) collects and disseminates cost data within its limited budget. To date, IHCCC has been more a data source rendering price comparisons for business enterprises than a policy think tank. Illinois is saddled with a hospital system that does not work well, and restrictive data policies (and academic researcher neglect) deny opportunities to identify specific flaws and test new directions. In the 1970s data on the hospital system were unavailable, but in the 1980s industry interests prevented their release to a larger public in forms usable to stimulate public policy reform.

Public Providers

The Chicago Department of Health (CDOH) clinics; Cook County Hospital (CCH), Oak Forest Hospital, and their affiliated ambulatory programs; the Cook County Department of Public Health; and the University of Illinois Hospitals and Clinics (UIH) constitute probably the most administratively backward and unintegrated urban public health care delivery system in the nation. Widely considered unresponsive, blatantly bureaucratic, and uncoordinated even at the most basic service level, together they control substantial jobs and public monies. The latter have been squandered in the face of mounting metropolitan health needs throughout the 1970s and 1980s and into the 1990s. Each unit claims shortages of funds, and administrative heads and political overlords have chosen not to make the necessary tough decisions to prioritize and to reallocate to achieve real public health improvements at the community level.

Four Veterans Administration hospitals serve the metropolitan region, each a province of one of the local medical schools: the University of Chicago Medical School, Northwestern, University of Illinois, and Loyola. These institutions, though they serve a significant number of indigent patients, have generally not been considered part of the public health delivery system by planners. Their administrative connections are purely through the medical school affiliations.

It is misleading to paint all public providers with a single stroke of the same brush. Although on the surface they share many of the same failings, closer analysis indicates that the scope and character of their respective situations do vary. An analysis of efficiency measures would yield very different results from Cook County Hospital and the University of Illinois Hospital. Other distinctions (e.g., credentials and competence of the management teams) can be drawn historically. Greater detail is thus helpful in evaluating past performances and assessing future potentials.

Of the FY 1990 Cook County budget of $1.7 billion, about 25 percent accounted for public health expenditures (criminal justice accounted for another two-thirds). The expenditure by the county government of over $280 million in local taxpayers' money can hardly signify an unwillingness to spend money; yet these funds were poorly concentrated on end-stage hospital services rather than on primary care and prevention. Decades of waste of Cook County Hospital monies for an eighty-year-old, inefficient, dying facility; perpetual construction contracts for its resuscitation; and phenomenal administrative waste and patronage all indicate the county's long-standing lack of proper stewardship over public monies supposedly dedicated for care of the poor and indigent. The 70 percent increase in health expenditures over the amount spent in 1985, with no commitment to improvements in services, echoes the same disregard for the Cook County taxpayer.

Likewise, reprioritization and strategic decisions for the optimal utilization of tax funding have not been major concerns of the state or the city. The legislature is currently subsidizing the University of Illinois Hospital (UIH) in the amount of $41.5 million a year on top of an accumulated deficit of over $12 million and despite its having the highest Medicaid ICARE reimbursement rate of any hospital in Illinois ($795 per day in 1989). The corporate funds of the city of Chicago allocated to its health department pale next to even medium-sized cities across the nation. The per capita spending for health programs of New York City, Los Angeles, and Philadelphia, among others, all rank higher. For the last five years, Chicago has given CDOH a 50 percent corporate allocation of $41.5 million (1990), with other funding for the city health program coming from state and federal sources.

The Chicago and Cook County Health Care Summit

In 1989 the Chicago and Cook County Health Care Summit was convened and given responsibility to draft legislation on how to improve the public provider situation in Cook County. To the extent that a power structure of local health care exists, it is best captured (without much grass-roots community input or involvement from nursing, pharmacy, dentistry, or other practitioners) in the sixty-some appointees to this deliberating body. Despite extensive media and community attention, the summit's recommendations (spring 1990) have never been implemented, although they would benefit the delivery system a great deal. However, the recommendations, overall, lacked courage, failed to challenge private interests, and did not criticize the public sector performance. Moreover, greater emphasis was placed on seeking financial relief from the state legislature than on initiatives for the Chicago and Cook County governments.

To a considerable extent, the focus of the summit members evolved from the historical thinking and advocacy of persons connected with a number of policy groups outside the public sector (e.g., the Health and Medicine Policy Research Group, the Metropolitan Planning Council, the Community Renewal Society, and numerous health professional groups). Unfortunately, these groups must collectively bear some responsibility for the failure of the summit to provide adequate representation to minority group members, users of services, women, nurses, and allied health professionals, among others.

A broader constituency of people working in the minority communities and public health care institutions has developed as a result of the lack of effective response from the political and bureaucratic leadership to the problems of indigent care delivery. Even some business leaders are now examining the situation post-summit, and alliances are likely to emerge among individuals acting in accordance with their basic human values rather than their organizational interests. Greater public sector responsiveness is more likely as advocates join forces to support a common, achievable agenda, and seek to overcome their political isolation.

The Acute-Care System

In 1980, sixty acute-care hospitals operated in Chicago; today there are fifteen fewer community institutions. The five academic medical centers now control over 20 percent of the beds, and another 30 percent are controlled by the eight other teaching hospitals.

As the area's third largest employer, the hospital sector in the Chicago region contains a larger proportion of facilities in the categories of 200–299 beds, 300–499 beds, and 500+ beds than the national norm. All hospital closures in Illinois since 1980 have involved facilities with fewer than 300 beds, except for St. Anne's, which was the largest institution (437 beds) in the nation to close during the 1980s.

In 1978 a total of 247 acute-care hospitals were operating in Illinois. Seventeen additional facilities were run by the Illinois Department of Mental Health and Developmental Disabilities to provide long-term acute and chronic services. (At the time, these seventeen were not accredited.) Over the 1980s, several hospitals outside of Chicago closed in the state.

During the decade, local and state hospital trends were generally reflective of the national situation, though Illinois still has more than the average number of available hospital beds per population. In 1979, Illinois hospitals had higher occupancy levels than hospitals in the United States as a whole, with occupancy levels in the metropolitan Chicago area much higher. The state exceeded the national averages in terms of inpatient days, admissions per 1,000 population, and average length of stay. At the end of the decade, these differences generally persisted. With an average of 4.91 beds per 1,000 population for the state in 1984, a growing surplus of beds became evident for the state and the city despite the decade's closures and the reduction in beds available at most institutions. These overall totals, however, obscure the serious restrictions on access to care of all kinds that certain communities have experienced at the same time that other communities remain overbedded.

More recently, Illinois has experienced a slightly lower hospital occupancy rate than the United States at large. Metro Chicago's rate remains higher than the state average but lower than the national rate. For the period 1978-1988, occupancy in the metro area declined by 19.6 percent, decreasing from 80 percent to 64.3 percent. In 1988, Chicago's occupancy rate of 63.1 percent was slightly lower than the statewide average, and its length of stay, 7.2 days, was slightly greater.

Percentage declines for admissions and inpatient days for metropolitan Chicago hospitals occurred over the decade. The decreases in utilization indicators for the late 1980s were generally smaller than the percentage changes before 1987. This phenomenon may indicate that the industry is leaner and more stable.

Data from the third quarter of 1989 indicated a continued downward slope, though at lower rates, for inpatient beds, total admissions, patient days, and average length of stay for the metro area. The occupancy rate increased to 67.9 percent for hospitals in the Chicago metro area and to 70.2 percent for those in Chicago proper. The latter figure reflects the impact of five hospital closures in 1987-1988, which accounted for a loss of 750 beds. It should be noted that occupancy in public hospitals is not significantly greater than in voluntary hospitals in the city, despite recent closures of community hospitals. One partial explanation might be that some former patients are not utilizing hospital care at prior levels; not much is known about the practice patterns in marginal or declining institutions, though several local observers have commented on the systemwide trend of reduced hospital use.

Table 3.1 presents a composite of hospital statistics by ownership for 1985 and 1988 for the city of Chicago, and Table 3.2 covers all of Cook County, including the city of Chicago. Absent from the tables are data on three local Veterans Administration hospitals (two in the city and the other in the suburbs) and two state mental hospitals (one in the city and one in the suburbs).

The public facilities covered in the tables include the Cook County Hospital and the University of Illinois Hospital, both in Chicago, as well as a county facility in Hinsdale, which was formerly used as a TB sanitorium, and the county's chronic disease facility, Oak Forest Hospital located in the suburbs, which now also provides some acute care.

The number of beds and admissions, average length of stay, and occupancy rate all declined over the decade for public hospitals, both city and suburban. For the 1985-1988 period, it should be noted that the two public suburban hospitals had significantly different service mixes than the metropolitan public hospitals. They provided a greater volume of chronic care, which is reflected in the longer ALOS. It should also be noted that the 1985 figures for beds, admissions, and average daily census for the suburban chronic disease hospital, Oak Forest, included the entire facility, but for 1988 only the acute beds were reported. This reporting discrepancy accounts for more than 80 percent of the decline in the number of beds and contributes heavily to the 60 percent drop in the ALOS among suburban public hospitals. Oak Forest operates 824 beds, of which approximately 150 are acute beds.

TABLE 3.1 Hospital Capacity and Utilization, Chicago, 1985 and 1988

Type of Ownership[a]	Year	Number of Hospitals	Number of Beds	Number of Admissions	Average Daily Census	Average Length of Stay (Days)	Occupancy (%)
Public[a]	1985	2	1,734	56,260	1,107	7.18	63.84
	1988	2	1,354	49,251	924	6.87	68.25
Percent Change		0	−21.91	−12.46	−16.53	−4.39	6.89
Voluntary	1985	53	15,348	492,321	10,236	7.59	66.69
	1988	44	12,589	402,812	9,414	7.64	66.83
Percent Change		−17	−17.98	−18.18	−17.81	0.73	0.21
Proprietary	1985	5	691	11,171	357	11.66	51.66
	1988	5	621	9,062	328	13.27	52.89
Percent Change		0	−10.13	−18.88	−8.00	13.72	2.37

[a]Data on two Veterans Administration hospitals and one state mental hospital are not included.

Source: AHA Hospital Statistics; IHCCCC Annual Price Survey, 1985, 1988.

TABLE 3.2 Hospital Capacity and Utilization, Cook County, 1985 and 1988

Type of Ownership	Year	Number of Hospitals	Number of Beds	Number of Admissions	Average Daily Census	Average Length of Stay (days)	Occupancy (%)
Public[a]	1985	4	2,910	60,653	2,115	12.73	72.68
	1988	4	1,641	51,192	1,103	7.89	68.47
Percent Change		0	−44.64	−15.60	−47.85	−38.04	−5.80
Voluntary	1985	77	24,494	820,846	16,786	7.46	68.53
	1988	68	21,106	711,577	14,308	7.36	67.79
Percent change		−11	−13.83	−13.31	−14.76	−1.41	−1.08
Proprietary	1985	9	1,432	24,836	912	13.40	63.68
	1988	9	1,343	25,976	880	12.40	65.54
Percent change		0	−6.22	4.59	−3.48	−7.46	2.92

[a]Data on three Veterans Administration hospitals and two state mental hospitals are not included.

Source: AHA Hospital Statistics; IHCCCC Annual Price Survey, 1985, 1988.

Among the three ownership categories, voluntary hospitals account for the vast majority of facilities (about 85 percent). In 1988, these sixty-eight facilities in Cook County had an average capacity of 310 beds and a range of 60 to 936 beds. The number of beds, number of admissions, ALOS, and occupancy all continued their downward slope over the decade among voluntary hospitals within the county. In contrast, for 1985 and 1988 the ALOS and occupancy remained virtually unchanged among voluntary hospitals within Chicago. The city's hospital closures may account in part for the magnitude of decline in the number of beds. However, admissions and average daily census show similar declines. This pattern suggests continuing changes in practice patterns toward less use of hospitals in general and perhaps the failure of some former patients to receive care after the hospital closures.

Although all suburban voluntary hospitals are general, short-term acute-care facilities, the city's voluntary hospitals include three children's hospitals in the county, two rehabilitation hospitals, and a psychiatric facility.

Of the nine proprietary hospitals in the county, more than half (five) are dedicated psychiatric facilities, which explains their longer ALOS. The range in size among proprietaries is 89 to 229 beds. Proprietary institutions exhibited gains in admissions (dramatically in the suburbs) and occupancy, accompanied by declines in number of beds and ALOS overall.

Hospital Closures

Hospital closures have become a very important issue in Chicago. Since 1980, twenty-two hospitals have closed in Illinois, fifteen in the city. Only two new hospitals opened in the state over the decade, both psychiatric facilities operated by national proprietary chains. Most closures came as a result of low reimbursement and declining occupancy, although several were victim to unique conditions.

In general, the fifteen hospitals that closed in Chicago (all but one since 1985) had a common geographic profile: They were located in underserved neighborhoods of greatest health care need. However, the closures of Lutheran General–Lincoln Park, Sheridan Road, and Mt. Sinai–North in 1989, and of Henrotin in 1986, were predominantly financial decisions based on competition in middle-class, overbedded neighborhoods. Henrotin, owned by Northwestern University, did serve a significant percentage of low-income patients from the nearby Cabrini-Greene Chicago Housing Project, confirming the hypothesis regarding the financial determinant for closure.

Closures not only severely affect the surrounding community economically but decrease general access to service outside the hospital (because, for example, they result in the subsequent relocation of physicians' offices, pharmacies, and other health and social service providers). The loss of jobs from a hospital closure is problematic, for even lower-paid nursing, housekeeping, and dietary workers who usually live (often as homeowners) in the served neighborhoods. A large percentage of such personnel find difficulty in securing comparable employment at comparable wage levels, if at all. Moreover, as shown by the recent closing of Central Community Hospital, pressures on other at-risk institutions are increased. In this case, the burden of Central Community's black patients was shifted to St. Bernard's, and Holy Cross took over responsibility for many of the displaced whites.

Not all closed hospitals in Chicago remain "dead capital, " that is, unused physical plants. Booth Hospital is being used by the Salvation Army as a homeless shelter. The closed Walther Memorial Hospital near Westtown has been purchased and converted to a psychiatric institution (called University Hospital) by a proprietary group associated with the Illinois School of Professional Psychology. The Frank Cuneo Facility has been turned into a Catholic boys residence as a joint venture with Columbus-Cuneo-Cabrini Medical Center and Maryville Academy. The Illinois Department of Drug and Alcohol Abuse is considering reopening the Mary Thompson Hospital for addicted pregnant women.

The St. Anne's plant on the Westside was purchased by Bethel New Life, a not-for-profit community corporation, for the purpose of setting up a long-term-care and residential facility. Another community-based provider, the Westside Holistic Health Center, now operates its former Professional Office Building, which has attracted a University of Illinois clinic, the Chicago Department of Health maternal-child station, and an assortment of other practitioners and agencies. Spokespersons for Bethel New Life have been quoted as saying they would be willing to have Cook County Hospital use the St. Anne's hospital facility as a decentralized unit because the Far Westside is underbedded and a large portion of Cook County Hospital's patients originate there. (A point of fact is that the corridor from the Near Westside through Austin contains one of the greatest concentrations of beds in the nation and, according to the Illinois Health Facilities Planning Board, has a sufficient number of beds for the population. The problem is the bed distribution and their overall service pattern. Beds are clustered at the Near Westside Medical Center, and they are chiefly high-tech beds, which are generally targeted to a much broader metro population. Ambulatory services, however, are absent in Westside communities.

On the South Side, the only black-founded hospital in the city, Provident Medical Center, was auctioned in 1989 by the U.S. Department of Housing and Urban Development. The governor eventually took title when the former president of the Cook County Board of Commissioners chose *not* to bid and a Black community group, the New Provident Community Organization, failed because it could not secure financing. The hospital has been given to Cook County to operate as a replacement facility for Cook County Hospital. About 42 percent of Cook County Hospital's patient population resides in South Side neighborhoods; many come, for example, from the Robert Taylor Homes, a Chicago Housing Authority structure of 29,000 persons. Over $30 million is needed to renovate the Provident facility, and the county's timetable for its opening has been postponed to late 1992.

Provident Hospital owed over $44 million in government funds when it closed in 1987. As a private hospital in a barren, impoverished area, Provident was never able to attract sufficient patients or admitting physicians and thus operated well below its 300-bed capacity and in the red. South Side black politics and intergovernmental discord confounded an earlier proposed takeover of this relatively new facility by the county.

In considering overall hospital failures in Chicago, the same pressures—declining occupancy, low Medicaid reimbursement, growing ranks of unsponsored patients, tight HMO/PPO negotiated rates, and regionally monitored payments by self-insured employers and commercial firms—that have stimulated corporate restructuring strategies among the more advantaged institutions also account for the distress of these health facilities. Based on financial ratios, several analysts estimate that up to seven more hospitals in the city remain at risk for closure (four on the Southwest Side alone). State of Illinois funds of $63 million became available in FY 1989 for institutions accumulating losses from serving large uninsured populations. For example, in 1988 Oak Park Hospital, owned by the Wheaton Franciscan Services, was considered to be the first candidate for failure among the near western suburban hospitals until a new, outside proprietary management team and additional Medicaid reimbursement under the disproportionate share program have enabled it to continue in operation.

A more critical determinant of hospital survival or failure may be community perceptions of quality of care. It is interesting to note that no hospitals relocated during the decade, although Rush-Sheraton is to undergo conversion to a rehabilitation facility. The parent Rush corporation is planning to build a 200-bed facility in the Southwest suburb of Tinley Park in the mid-1990s.

Restructuring Strategies

In conjunction with closures, a dramatic restructuring occurred in the local hospital industry. Internal reorganization accompanied a greater concentration of ownership and management among local/regional systems. Subsidiary ventures blossomed, especially among larger institutions. Hospitals may have as many as five to eight subsidiaries under a corporate shell, often hidden from its full board of trustees, competitors, and regulators. For example, Rush-Presbyterian–St. Luke's has a set of health plans (Anchor HMO, Rush-ACCESS, Rush-CONTRACT, and Rush-OCCUPATIONAL HEALTH) and extensive real estate holdings in housing, retail, and hotel ventures.

Useful for public relations in supporting claims of government underfunding of patient care, such investment strategies have kept overall corporate margins in the black for some hospitals facing the demographic squeeze on paying patients. Rumors occasionally circulate that certain hospital administrators and board members personally profit from such business endeavors that are beyond the original hospital mission. Concerns over joint ventures with a hospital's medical staff have also drawn local scrutiny, following the debate in professional journals.

An increase in the number of specialized hospital beds was accompanied by the regionalization of services. By 1987, acute care hospitals in Illinois had set up forty-one (twenty-six in Chicago) alcoholism and substance-abuse units; fifteen (nine in the city) rehabilitation units; six (three in the city) burn units; and nine (all in Chicago) pediatric ICUs.

With regard to changes in mission, a Chicago Health Executive Forum study in 1989 found that metro hospitals have perceptibly shifted to a business orientation. Its analysis of mission and financial statements revealed that area hospitals did not pay $261.4 million in federal and state income taxes and property and sales taxes because of their nonprofit status. Moreover, they realized $190.7 million from their ability to borrow in tax-exempt capital markets. Thus, between 1985 and 1987 these so-called not-for-profit hospitals realized more than $450 million in tax subsidies but provided only about half of this amount ($215 million) in charity care to the uninsured. At least as expressed in their mission statements, suburban hospitals placed greater emphasis on public service, although their indigent case loads are lower than those of the inner-city hospitals due to their locations.

The issue of mission also surfaced when the University of Illinois Board of Trustees altered its hospital's tradition of serving the poor and needy. Public outcry accompanied the board's decision in 1987 to close the hospital and clinics to patients who were not sponsored or could not pay. Long before this, most private hospitals in Chicago had taken direct actions to limit indigent care, from outright "dumping" of patients to Cook County's emergency room to closing or downsizing their outpatient departments. Although ambulatory statistics at Chicago hospitals exhibited phenomenal growth over the decade, much of this increase occurred because the hospitals targeted paying clienteles in preference to residents in their surrounding poor communities. In fact, significant "demarketing" of Medicaid and indigent populations took place in response to several state cutbacks and the overall increase in the number of the uninsured.

Ambulatory Care

Chicago has seen significant growth in ambulatory-care services. The institution of the prospective payment system (PPS) encouraged a national shift to outpatient care. The restrictions of private insurance companies on reimbursement for inpatient services also contributed. Area hospitals diversified their outpatient services to capture new markets and to retain the paying segments of their current ones. Limited reimbursement still plagues many ambulatory services, particularly when established outpatient and emergency services are in demand by inner-city Medicaid recipients. For some suburban hospitals, there have been increases in intensive technological procedures performed in out-of-hospital settings, often set up as joint ventures with physician groups. Reliable data on the extent of these activities are not available.

The dominance of hospitals and their density in Chicago may account for the paucity of free-standing ambulatory ventures by entrepreneurial physicians, such as are seen in other places around the country. There have been some new ventures, particularly on the Northwest Side, but these seem confined to specialty practices (e.g.; ophthalmology, liposuction, and the hernia and hemorrhoid trade). Reportedly, only two physician groups own CAT scanners. Despite many reductions in hospital outpatient departments since the mid-1980s (moves principally made to reduce the number of Medicaid and uninsured patients), hospitals still control the vast majority of ambulatory surgery and most of the extensive equipment-related procedures.

Other ambulatory developments include a broad array of incentives to attract and retain physician loyalty. For example, physicians have been offered full-time faculty practice plans by the academic medical centers; new office buildings have been erected at community hospitals to encourage professional bonding to the institution. More recently, same-day surgery units have been established, often off the hospital campus. Other joint ventures for high-tech equipment are commonplace. Two additional means hospitals have used to ensure continuing admission streams are the purchase of physician practices in attractive communities and HMO/PPO diversification.

Emergency Care

Once known nationally for its advanced planning for emergency medical services, Illinois now has little in which to take pride in this area. The

Chicago trauma network has undergone a period of near shambles organizationally. Established by the Chicago Department of Health in 1986,
the trauma network included at that time ten hospitals designated to provide adult trauma services and six to provide pediatric trauma services. In
1988, the trauma care system handled more than 1,500 cases, 312 of which
ended in deaths; the number of cases was up from 1,346 in 1987, 322 of
which ended in deaths. The survival rate of 76.1 percent among severely
injured Level I victims in 1987 and 78 percent in 1988 compared favorably
with other urban systems in the nation.

In May 1988, the University of Chicago (UC) dropped out of the trauma
network, citing insufficient reimbursement, and was followed by Weiss
Memorial Hospital in the North Lakeshore area. The withdrawal of Weiss
was not overly problematic because Northwestern Hospital was still accessible to most trauma patients in the area. However, the UC pullout left
Michael Reese as the only South Side trauma facility. In November 1988,
administrators at Reese announced that it too would leave, but then rescinded their decision. Loyola, in suburban Maywood, dropped out of the
city network in 1989. In February 1990, Reese officially withdrew, leaving
no South Side hospital within Chicago's borders in the trauma network.
Christ Hospital and Medical Center in western suburban Oak Lawn now
assumes the huge South Side load.

Christ Hospital, a participant in both the state and city trauma networks, saw dramatic increases in the number of trauma patients between
its first year in the network and 1989. In 1989, 1,153 Level I trauma patients
were admitted, up from 265 in 1987. Many trauma victims are uninsured
or Medicaid recipients or have private insurance that does not pay full
fees. A regionalization plan by the city designated the relatively distant
Cook County, Northwestern, and Mount Sinai hospitals to receive more of
the South Side trauma load, thereby relieving Christ Hospital of part of
the burden. Survival rates may decline from the rates calculated for 1987–
1988 because of the smaller number of hospitals in the network, but no
point within city limits reportedly exceeds 30 minutes' travel time to a
Level I center. In fact, according to the American College of Surgeons
standards for recommended patient volume, Chicago needs only between
three and five centers citywide.

Complicating the problems of the trauma system is the severe ambulatory-care gridlock of Medicaid and uninsured patients. Hospital emergency rooms sometimes face patient overloads, and when they do, ambulance drivers divert patients to hospitals with available capacity,
"bypassing" institutions with no room. As a result of inadequate means of
providing primary care, thirteen city hospital emergency rooms went on
ER bypass in December 1989, when monitored beds became full. Partly

due to an influenza epidemic, this phenomenon again indicates the need for more effective planning and coordination within the delivery system.

Competition and Financing

As discussed, the dominance of academic medical centers and teaching hospitals in the acute-care system gives the local health care industry a unique character. New technology acquisitions are not, however, confined solely to these larger players. It is reported that high-tech medicine is more broadly diffused than might be expected. The teaching hospitals and community hospitals faced much less intense competition in the Chicago area in the 1980s than in other areas of the United States even though Reagan pro-competitive policies reigned ideologically among hospital executives there as elsewhere. As total revenues for most private institutions grew appreciably over the decade, a certain midwestern organizational individualism to "do your own thing and let the other guy alone" may have kept outright conflicts to a minimum. Likewise, the failure of academic medical centers to be more of a political force in health care may be partially attributed to the same cultural climate. Nevertheless, the past few years of hospital closures and new grabs for increased market shares by the larger systems may be altering this relatively non-competitive atmosphere with quite different outcomes for the immediate future.

The local hospital industry remains viable, but it is leaner now. From 1985 on, there has been little new capital investment in physical plants by Chicago hospitals. Since the Illinois Health Facilities Planning Board raised the floor for a certificate of need to $2 million per project, it is difficult to keep track of what might be called "minor" renovations, conversions, and introductions of new equipment. As an indicator of the restrictions being placed on new acquisitions to upgrade quality, certain hospitals have replenished rather old and outdated technology by purchasing used, discounted equipment from hospitals that have closed. Financial constraints in certain Chicago institutions may be curtailing needed modernization.

Changes in health care financing over the last decade significantly affected Chicago. Whereas the advent of prospective payment under Medicare in 1983 brought benefits to several teaching hospitals (as well as a number of proprietary home health care firms), more than a few community hospitals lost their ability to reap high profits from the over-sixty-five population. If the ICARE program had not simultaneously jarred these vulnerable institutions, their situation may not have become critical. Implementation of the DRGs coincided with the initiation of the state's ICARE program in 1984. With private insurance companies resisting cost-shifting and numerous larger firms instituting self-insurance, and with purchaser monitoring of hospital charges, hospital revenues tightened severely. This fiscal squeeze has surely not ended.

The financial status of more than a few institutions remains precarious. Hospitals that did not react quickly after 1983 with cost-cutting preparations after the 1983 implementation of PPS are among them. It was reported that the chairman of the House Ways and Means Committee, Representative Daniel Rostenkowski, initially aided Illinois hospitals in securing favorable payment rates. However, Medicare payments for Chicago hospital stays are now at the national DRG rates. The 1991 Bush administration budget for Medicare threatens to cut previously anticipated inpatient revenues for metro area hospitals by an estimated $77 million, a move that will hit the teaching institutions the hardest.

With regard to Medicaid, it has been reported community hospitals in Chicago are reimbursed by the IDPA for about 30–40 percent of the patients they discharge (in contrast to numbers as low as 6 percent for suburban proprietary institutions). For private academic health centers (AHCs), the number is approximately 10 percent. Because patients whose care is reimbursed by the Medicaid program are generally treated less intensively than others, they tend to have shorter average lengths of stay. Smaller community (usually religious) hospitals apparently sustain greater Medicaid patient utilization, either in conformity with their mission to their surrounding community or due to their locked-in location. This trend represents a change from the early 1980s. The Medicaid ICARE program reallotted days to lower-cost institutions after 1985, and partly due to competitive responses, the AHCs have secured the better insured patients.

Recent payments for Medicaid recipients under ICARE are claimed by the IHA to be near 68 cents per dollar billed for inpatient care; IDPA payment delays are commonplace and significant. State comparisons of Medicaid usually rank the Illinois program thirty-ninth in per recipient expenditures, even though the number of recipients (1.043 million in 1988) and total expenditures ($1. 8 billion) rank eighth and seventh, respectively. To demonstrate the extent of underpayment to hospitals by Illinois Medicaid, the state's per diem payment in 1989 was reported to be 55 percent that of Blue Cross ($541 compared to $979) for metropolitan teaching hospitals and 58 percent that of Blue Cross for nonteaching community hospitals ($349 compared to $598).

In addition, local hospitals have faced other pressures for financial contraction. Several HMOs and PPOs have exacted "bargains" on their inpatient bills; hospital administrators claim the necessity of holding onto certain HMO contracts for the sake of occupancy, even though the hospitals do not realize much profit on these patients.

Increases in hospital charges have been reported by the Illinois Health Care Cost Containment Council, which has published price data for the 235 hospitals in Illinois since the mid-1980s. For 1988, the average charge for a patient in an Illinois hospital at discharge was $5,466—a 10.2 percent increase from the preceding year—with an average daily charge of $841. These charges may be compared to those of the Chicago metropolitan area. For Health Service Area (HSA) Six (Chicago), the amounts were $7,384 and $1, 026, respectively, and for HSA Seven (Suburban Cook and DuPage counties), they were $5,950 and $888, respectively.

Given all of the factors that have been discussed, it is estimated that 75 percent of Chicago area hospitals lose money on patient service operations, with more than a few consuming their equity as they are threatened by possible closure. Hence, hospitals see investments, joint ventures, and charitable support as necessary for maintaining their bottom lines at fiscal year end.

Alternative Delivery Systems

Alternative delivery systems grew rapidly in Illinois in the 1980s, especially in the metropolitan region. Although President Richard Nixon's HMO strategy had stimulated the growth of HMOs in several other states, by 1978 only 1 percent of Illinois' population were enrolled in health maintenance organizations. Thereafter, enrollment began to escalate, but since the early 1980s the rate of increase in Illinois has slowed considerably. The number of HMO firms in operation rose from eleven in 1980 to forty-six in 1992. Before five went out of business, the first doing so in 1987, a clear majority were for-profit.

In the Chicago area, enrollment rose from 200,000 to nearly 1.5 million as several new firms entered the scene. In 1986-1987 there was a 21 percent increase in enrollees, down from a 98 percent increase in 1983-1984. This trend is generally consistent with national trends; for the United States as a whole, enrollments leveled off at 30 million according to Interstudy. Observers claim that the local Chicago market is now showing signs of "maturity." About 26 percent of Chicagoans—the high watermark for HMO enrollment in Chicago—were enrolled near the end of the 1980s.

Particularly in the metropolitan region, the growth of HMOs occurred simultaneously with a decline in hospital utilization over the decade. Hospital executives claimed that competing for HMO contracts complicated their crimped profits from their paying patients, but the added business nonetheless maintained occupancy. One analyst in 1988 described the situation as "hospitals complain, but they don't scream." Problems arise in paying for trauma, spinal cord injury, perinatal and other high-cost admissions.

As is the case nationally, the narrowing trend in HMOs faces a 1990s shakeout in the area. Of the Chicago-based HMO firms, most are under-capitalized, and all but one experienced losses in 1989. The once obtrusive marketing campaigns across the Chicago landscape and airwaves are vir-tually gone. In the mid-1980s, Maxicare pulled out of the Medicare mar-ket, a move that had a significant impact on the Illinois health care mar-ket. Because most Chicago-based HMOs are organized in the IPA model, they are vulnerable to physician withdrawals as doctors realize they can make more money and are subject to less financial risk with PPOs.

Both regional and national for-profit HMOs have concentrated on at-tracting employed, relatively healthy (and thus profitable) patients. In 1980, fewer than 280,000 people were enrolled in the state's seven HMOs; by 1987, forty-six HMOs served nearly 1,378,000 Illinois citizens. Of these, 61 percent were for-profit entities. Several locally owned for-profit HMOs of less than reputable quality sought IDPA Medicaid contracts.

The accounting firm of Touche Ross claims that 85 percent of the HMO business in Illinois is concentrated in fourteen firms with more than 30,000 enrollees each. Those firms have been facing a decline in profitability: Only six showed a positive net income in 1987. About 55 percent of the metro Chicago HMOs (of a total of twenty-nine) showed losses on reve-nue of $1.8 billion in 1987. All fourteen of the larger Illinois firms had losses of $31 million in 1987 (compared to profits of $5 million in 1986 and $22 million in 1985). What may account for this decline in revenue is the fact that the firms did not increase their premiums between 1985 and 1987 due to the competitiveness of the market. During those years, a few firms sought to increase their enrollment and market share at the expense of profitability.

The medical loss ratio rose to 91 percent in 1987; it had been 85 percent in 1985. Physician utilization and other outpatient services have not been easily controlled in recent years, mostly due to the IPA mode. Physician visits more than doubled in 1987, averaging 4. 8 encounters per enrollee. Although there was a large growth over the last half of the 1980s in HMO participation, a few firms have faced high physician turnover and losses. The annualized hospital inpatient utilization dropped from 460 to 400 days per 1,000 enrollees during 1985–1987. For the latter year, the re-ported average length of stay for an HMO hospital patient was 4.5 days, compared to 7 days for all inpatients in Chicago. Administrative expenses for HMOs remained stable at about the national average of 11–12 percent. Premiums, however, rose in 1988–1989 as HMO firms attempted to regain profit positions, and more aggressive utilization management was insti-tuted.

Aside from the HMOs operated by the commercial insurance compa-nies (e.g, CIGNA, MetLIFE, Prucare, and Aetna), provider-sponsored

HMOs dominate in membership totals. The largest, HMO Illinois, which is run by Blue Cross/Blue Shield of Illinois, had in 1989 over 300,000 members. (Blue Cross also owns the largest PPO, Participating Provider Option, which had 526,066 enrollees in 1988.) In addition, there are a university-affiliated HMO (at the University of Illinois at Chicago) and a union-sponsored HMO.

A hybrid form of prepaid health care is now appearing as certain local HMOs are also offering HMO/ASOs (administrative services only) contracts. These HMO/ASOs provide utilization management for self-funded employers who take on the insurance risk themselves. It is not clear how such arrangements will compete with PPOs in their evolution in the metropolitan area.

Because of the short history of the other new organizational forms in the metropolitan region, less data have accumulated describing their development. The urgent care center, or urgi-center, which is a free-standing emergency center, arose in the late 1970s in the form of group physician practices operating on an extended-hour basis. Dr. Ned Flashner began a chain of suburban urgent care centers, mainly in the collar county area, and later sold them to Humana Corporation as the nucleus of its MedFirst network. It was subsequently sold to its participating physicians and other investors when the Humana Care Plus operation faced huge losses in Illinois. A number of hospitals have also opened or affiliated with free-standing urgi-centers.

Another new provider form was the ambulatory surgical treatment center (AST), or surgi-center. These free-standing entities were typically started by physicians to capture the estimated 40 percent of surgeries that can be performed on an outpatient basis. Of note in Illinois are the eye and liposuction clinics, which both advertise heavily. Surgi-centers are licensed by the Illinois Department of Public Health, but urgi-centers, the bulk of which are in the suburbs, are not.

Along with the formation of multihospital corporations, attempts at creating organized systems out of these new organizational forms helped reshape the metro health care arena over the decade. Most of these efforts laid the groundwork for potential combinations in the future. The "local market" orientation, which is spoken about these days as some national health care corporations flounder in their broader strategies, has been in evidence in Chicago, at least since 1985.

Preferred provider organizations stand more readily to gain in market share in the 1990s. They have studiously enlisted various providers under their financing umbrellas. As the subscriber base for PPOs has grown, hospitals in need of occupancy and medical groups willing to discount their fees for increased volume (ranging up to 30 percent) have signed up in large numbers. In 1988, about thirty-one PPOs operated in metro Chicago and fifteen operated in other parts of Illinois, for an approximate total of forty-six. Most had under 25,000 enrollees. Reliable information on PPOs is unavailable because, unlike HMOs, they are not required to report to the Illinois Department of Insurance. (The MCHC gathers much more incomplete and much less detailed data on PPOs than it does on HMOs.)

Most locally-based PPOs are provider-sponsored, but observers see more insurance company PPOs becoming dominant (contracting with smaller providers for cost savings and locational advantages, i.e., suburban locations). The CIGNA purchase of Equicor extends a vast market for this firm in Illinois. In addition, more employers are seeking to deal with only one vendor for a "triple option," so major insurers may also gain in market share in this way. Some expect managed care to move toward EPOs (exclusive provider organizations), in which all employees of a contracting firm are restricted to a preselected set of physicians based on utilization controls.

Physicians, Nurses, and Other Health Professionals

The number of health professionals in Illinois and Chicago increased dramatically during the 1980s due to extensive educational programs in the state. The American Hospital Association's *Hospital Statistics, 1987* Edition reported that there were 190,210 hospital personnel in Illinois in 1987, making hospitals the fifth largest employer in Illinois. Figures increased in all categories through 1990, and the nonhospital-based health workers add substantially to these numbers.

Because of its medical teaching and research programs, Illinois has long been a net exporter of physicians, the fourth highest in the nation. With eight medical schools (including several campuses of the state university system outside Chicago), a large number of physicians are trained each year, as are a wide variety of nursing specialists, pharmacists, dentists, and allied health professionals.

For 1985, the inequitable distribution of physicians in Illinois (as elsewhere) was most noticeable downstate, where there was an estimated shortage of 346 primary care physicians. The shortage resulted in a physician/population ratio of 1:3,500 in all designated underserved areas. This deficit is considerably more severe than that found in shortage areas in Indiana, Michigan, Minnesota, Ohio, and Wisconsin.

In 1980, there were 5,157 licensed physicians with Chicago addresses (the figure is unadjusted for practice settings). Although the primary care physician/population ratio for the city was 1:2,242 in 1975—not an inadequate number then—severe service gaps existed, as they still do (although now exacerbated) in the West and South sides of the city. Forty-three of

Chicago's seventy-seven community areas are underserved according to national criteria. Whereas the city as a whole has a physician/population ratio of about 1:850 persons, the ratio in shortage areas may be as low as 1:16,000 or 17,000. There are only 350 black and Hispanic physicians out of a total of 9,500 medical practitioners. Following the national trend, more women are entering medical practice, most often in salaried positions or part-time.

Within this medical mecca, the significant shortages of primary care physicians are particularly problematic in a number of Chicago neighborhoods. Because of high malpractice insurance costs, it is reported that several obstetricians have left their practices. Probably due to hospital closings and low Medicaid payments, physician relocations out of the South and West sides appear to have taken place in the last half of the decade, though the evidence is anecdotal. The Chicago area remains a medical magnet for foreign medical graduates, some of whom get their start in Medicaid practices before moving to more affluent areas.

More recently, Medicaid participating physicians (many without hospital affiliations), the seven Chicago Department of Health Centers, and the federally funded "Section 330" community health centers have filled some of the gaps in primary care. (Although providers in the latter two categories are most visible, private physicians in small group practices may deliver the largest share of patient visits.) Nevertheless, access problems within the inner city remain critical due to patients' inability to pay, waiting times for appointments, and cultural and language barriers especially for Hispanics and Southeast Asians. Other private group practices have expanded greatly in the metropolitan area in the 1980s, but these have catered to the more affluent. The incentives for these private groups have been the financial advantages, the ability to share medical equipment and facilities, and the ease with which large numbers of prospective patients can be attracted.

The medical school class size for private institutions has remained generally stable. However, the University of Illinois administration sought to cut its incoming class size by 25 percent in 1988, but it settled for 15 percent due to faculty resistance. Reports indicate declining applications at all schools, and at the University of Illinois, quality standards are now a concern. Because of faculty turmoil and losses, the highly publicized debacle in securing an affiliation with Michael Reese Hospital, and the University of Illinois Hospital's financial plight, the medical residency programs failed to match in 1988 and 1989. For the University of Illinois, as well as a few other residency programs across Chicago's teaching hospitals, there have been both reductions in and outright elimination of some of the specialty residencies.

The dental schools at Northwestern, Loyola, and the University of Illinois at Chicago faced all the problems that confronted other dental schools in the nation during the 1980s. Their graduates flocked to the suburban markets, generally leaving the black, Hispanic, Asian, and poorer elderly—the populations most in need of dental services—without care. Enrollments dropped dramatically in all schools. Between 1986 and 1988 the number of entering students at the University of Illinois decreased by 41 percent to a total of 80 students with a drop to 60 students expected soon. Enrollments at Loyola and Northwestern decreased about 50 percent each during that period—to 75 and 66 freshmen, respectively. Admission standards have lessened and attrition rates climbed. Starting salaries for new graduates remained constant and in some areas actually declined in the late 1980s as a result of practitioner competition.

The state's only college of pharmacy and its school of public health, both at the University of Illinois at Chicago, grew in size across the decade and did not encounter a dearth of student applicants. Pharmacy in particular is a financially rewarding field, with starting salaries at chain drugstores near $50,000 annually. Hospitals encounter a shortage of pharmacists, however. Public health and health policy and planning students generally find jobs in public- and community-based health and human services agencies, as well as in the numerous national health organizations in the metropolitan area.

The 1986 biennial survey of Illinois registered nurses conducted by the University of Illinois at Chicago College of Nursing found 84 percent of licensed RNs working in nursing positions, compared to 81 percent in 1984. About 53 percent were working full-time, compared to 56 percent in 1984. Twenty-six percent were working part-time, up 1.5 percent from two years earlier. About 1 percent were not working but were seeking RN employment, 3 percent were not working in nursing, and another 4 percent were over sixty-five years of age. Approximately 1.5 percent were not working but were enrolled in a formal academic program. The pattern was reported to be consistent across the Illinois health service areas. The findings suggest that there is almost no nursing unemployment in Illinois and that there are almost no untapped nursing personnel resources.

Of the nurses, 48 percent hold diplomas, 22 percent hold associate degrees and 30 percent hold baccalaureate or higher nursing degrees. Almost 60 percent of those working hold staff nurse positions, and 25 percent more are in management roles. Over 66 percent work in hospitals, 8 percent in nursing homes, 5.2 percent in doctors' offices, 4.7 percent in public and community health, and another 4.3 percent in clinics. The 1988 survey found 86 percent of licensed nurses actively working as nurses, representing the highest level of employment in any female career choice in Illinois. The proportion of nurses working in hospitals dropped to 62.5

percent, and the proportion of those under thirty dropped from 21.7 to 18.4 percent.

The nursing shortage is not as critical in Illinois as it is in many other regions of the country. Nevertheless, only a handful of hospitals can get all the nurses they want. The high-tech specialties hold more status within the profession; other positions (for instance, general med-surg nursing for chronically ill geriatric patients) may be harder to fill. The "burnout" areas of emergency room, operating room, and intensive care nursing also face constant turnover. Hospital strategy has shifted from nurse recruitment to nurse retention; however, some evening and night shift jobs remain unfilled at most institutions.

Given this situation, the business of the private registries, as elsewhere, is booming. Several hospitals negotiate volume discounts for agency nurses, and a few nursing departments have set up their own in-house pools in defense. The differential wage rates for these part-time agency nurses are significant, but most institutions have worked with this condition long enough to gain some measure of predictability in staffing.

The Illinois Nurses Association addressed the shortage issue, and hospitals are responding—though unevenly—with career ladders, job enrichment, burnout seminars, and so forth. Illinois nurses have complained about the hospital workload; about the higher proportion of patients who are generally sicker, and about shortages of ancillary personnel. The association reported a vacancy rate for hospital nursing personnel statewide of 5.2 percent in 1985. This figure jumped to 9. 7 percent in 1987, but in 1989 and continuing through 1990 it remained lower than prevailing national rates of 13–15 percent. There are 110,000 licensed RNs in the state. Seventy thousand of the 92, 000 who are working are employed by Illinois hospitals. Fewer than 19,000 first-year students are enrolled in nursing programs today.

Although not severe, the nursing shortage in metropolitan Chicago is reflected in rising vacancy rates (from 3.9 percent in 1984 to 9.6 percent in 1988), alleviated at some institutions only by agency placements and foreign nursing graduates. Persistent recruitment campaigns indicate the reality that hospitals, particularly those in the inner city, face difficult times. For the city, the resulting stress on hospitals, as well as on patients, is reported to be acute for many specialties, from trauma and burn at Cook County Hospital to most categories at the University of Illinois Hospital and to other clinical areas at many community hospitals.

Even the Chicago Department of Health cannot recruit sufficient public health nurses (PHNs) for essentially nine-to-five jobs. The salary scale for PHNs is lower than that for hospital floor nurses and is far less than what PHNs can earn in occupational health settings in private industry. Even though the city's pay scale for PHNs is negotiated through collective bargaining with the Illinois Nurses Association, working conditions at the clinics are a disincentive for the more mobile younger nurses today to opt for a lifetime career in these settings.

Many suburban institutions have been able to get by much better thus far. Flexible programs have been initiated, starting salaries have been raised, and the upper salary limits are considerably higher than in the past. Nevertheless, there remains generalized dissatisfaction among nurses with working conditions across the range of metro Chicago health providers. Rising patient care needs, the intensity of care required due to increased levels of acuity, and problems with advancement in salary and rank are still said to be critical. Lack of autonomy within the bureaucratic structure and overriding physician prerogatives are increasingly cited as problems needing remedial action if the nursing situation is to be improved in the 1990s.

Personnel shortages in certain other categories are equally acute. The Metropolitan Chicago Healthcare Council's biennial compensation survey in 1988 found the highest vacancy rates among health care personnel for physical therapists (15.4 percent); radiologic technicians (6 percent); cardiac technicians (5.5 percent); and pharmacists (5.1 percent). Personnel shortages for pharmacists in community practice as well as for dentists, podiatrists, and chiropractors were reported for the more economically depressed neighborhoods.

More severe health worker shortages for the Chicago area are predicted for the 1990s due to a compression of the ranks of high school candidates for health careers, smaller cohorts of college-age students, and withdrawal of qualified professionals, particularly nurses, from the health care field.

Long Term Care

Long term care (LTC) has not been a prominent policy issue in Illinois; it fails to get much attention even among health professionals. Media coverage of LTC issues during the 1980s was sporadic, but lack of coverage does not mean that major reform is not needed. The Governor's Conference on Long Term Care in 1988 started the process toward policy reform, but much remains problematic. Compared to the acute care system, LTC has seen little pressure for action outside of a few constituent groups (mainly the Illinois Citizens for Better Care, which has campaigned successfully for some changes) and some additional support from mental health groups and groups for the aged. The Better Government Association published a consumer guide to LTC facilities in Cook County in 1990 to mark its beginning support for health and human service agencies.

The federal mandate for nursing home residents with developmental disabilities (DD) effective in FY 1987-1988 catalyzed much action. Continuing pressure for creating community-integrated settings for the large numbers of these residents who must be discharged is needed because the state has not had favorable experience in such matters. As a result of the mandate, a substantial proportion of nursing home beds, which were occupied by DD patients, have been cleared: Over 6,000 adults and 1,500 children with DD problems in Illinois nursing homes were targeted.

It is not yet known how such massive deinstitutionalization will affect the nursing home industry over the next several years. The declined occupancy and lower utilization stays could lead to closures, which would affect access in certain areas. Another scenario might be that the greater number of available beds could lead to a greater acceptance of AIDS patients by nursing homes. However, if beds open up for patients with more severe clinical (and much more costly) problems, pressures will mount for increased reimbursements from public, as well as private, sources.

Generally, patients in the Chicago area are most in need of subacute-care facilities, and some hospitals have been converting their unused capacity for this purpose. In fact, several hospitals are operating "nursing home" wings, having secured approval for long-term bed conversions from the Illinois Health Facilities Planning Board. Other hospitals "disguise" long-term beds as chronic care units or hospices. Transfers to such units rarely come from outside institutions.

As already implied, AIDS patients are reportedly not getting into many nursing homes and are thus staying in the more costly hospital setting. A few voluntary community efforts, such as Chicago House are providing AIDS patients with housing that includes some care assistance, but none of these community efforts are certified as skilled nursing services. Oak Forest Hospital, part of the county system in the far south suburbs, has several beds allocated for AIDS patients, but they more than likely are filled only from Cook County Hospital transfers. The overall problem of inadequate care for AIDS patients throughout the metro area will likely complicate the existing burdens on health facilities in the public sector. The dominance of the for-profit sector over the long-term industry in Illinois, the lack of private insurance coverage for LTC, and the significant underpayment by Medicaid make it unlikely that the new clientele (AIDS, Alzheimer's, and technology-dependent patients) will receive proper care.

In Chicago, the stock of beds for long term care is inadequate but is reportedly not in "crisis" with regard to general placement from hospitals, given the way the overall system operates. This may be partly due to the provision by the 1988 Medicare amendments of payment for five months for hospital-discharged patients with nasogastric (NG) tubes, intravenous, narcotics administration, broken hips, and colostomies. Supplemental Security Income (SSI) applications are often taken in the case of patients without funds, and a few nursing homes have been accepting such transfers if they are given a month's deposit by the family. Certain sections of the city are almost completely without nursing homes providing skilled nursing care.

The Illinois Department of Public Aid pays very little to nursing homes. (Reimbursement was at the rate of $36.70 per day in 1988 for intermediate and skilled nursing care, but that figure has increased somewhat since then.) As a result, a few desertions by the national corporate nursing home chains occurred over the last half of the past decade. Nearly 57 percent of LTC residents are under Medicaid reimbursement, even though the amount falls short of the median rate for care in Illinois of $57 per day (1988). In 1985 the State introduced a Quality Incentive Program (QUIP) to reward Medicaid providers who demonstrate improvements in nursing care. The program pays up to one dollar per day more than the standard rate, in 1988 totaling $15 million in IDPA outlays. Nursing home complaints about the program's required documentation have led to some reductions in the paperwork.

Hospital social workers speak openly about the quality trade-offs and problems with staff responsiveness at many local nursing homes. There have been allegations of staff shortages; low wage LPNs and nurse aides dominate, with very few RNs among the typical staff. In 1987 and 1988, the Illinois Department of Health found final or pending Type B violations (threats to health and safety) in twenty of the 274 licensed nursing homes in Cook County (60 percent are for-profit entities) .

The Illinois Department of Public Aid funds 56,000 persons, the majority of whom are over sixty-five years of age, housed in 860 LTC facilities in Illinois. More than $500 million are expended for their care, about one third of the state Medicaid budget. The federal portion of the Illinois Medicaid program is only 50 percent.

According to the Illinois Department of Public Aid, the number of skilled nursing care patient days declined from nearly 5 million in 1985 to less than 3 million in 1988, whereas intermediate care patient days edged up from over 15 million to approximately 18 million in 1988. In 1988, the number of licensed beds in the state was 108,333, over 90,000 of which were skilled or intermediate care beds.

Illinois manages the largest statewide home and community-based Medicaid waiver program in the United States. The state obtained a waiver for elderly, physically disabled, DD, and technology-dependent children for 15,000 Medicaid eligible persons annually.

Home care agencies have flourished in Chicago, but they serve exclusively paying patients. Home care remains a cottage industry, with

Upjohn a major player, together with several local for-profit firms. The severe competition for paying patients led the Visiting Nurse Association of Chicago to alter its mission in the 1980s; it now limits services to nonpaying clientele. Neither the county nor the city health department has mounted programs to fill the void for those without home health care coverage.

Hospice service organizations in the community abound, but these are mostly small, grass-roots professional efforts, with a growing number of hospital-based units for the patients of their staff physicians. Although the hospice benefit was granted under Medicare in 1984, these services are constrained due to physician hesitation in referral. An active voluntary association in Illinois promoted the hospice idea and resisted the intrusion of the nation's only for-profit hospice, which has now penetrated the Illinois market.

Upon first examination of available data, long-term health care in Illinois would appear *not* to follow the national trend toward absorption into the corporate sector. In 1987, for-profit long-term care facilities in the state accounted for 62.7 percent of all beds in Illinois, down approximately 7.2 percent from the 1981 figure. This decline occurred despite an overall increase in the number of long-term beds; the loss of for-profit beds and facilities was more than offset by an increase in not-for-profits. These statistics suggest that vigorous enforcement of standards by the Illinois Department of Public Health may have led to the closure or sale of certain for-profit facilities and that proprietary firms may have decided against constructing new (replacement) beds in certain areas of Illinois.

Illinois nursing home capacity more than doubled between 1971 and 1980, from 44,000 to 93,000 beds, as the proportion of those sixty-five and older rose from 9.8 to 11.0 percent of the population. Utilization of nursing homes by the mentally disabled increased dramatically over this time also. The number of patient days increased from 14 million in 1970 to over 30 million in 1981, with average occupancy hovering over 90 percent.

For 1988, 57 percent of the 980 licensed facilities in the state were proprietary, 36 percent were not-for-profit and 5 percent were public. In that year, there were a total of 108,405 licensed nursing home beds and 6,878 unlicensed beds in the state. The annual length of stay over the five-year period from 1984 to 1988 was relatively stable for intermediate care facilities, but the median SNF length of stay has declined steadily, from forty-four days to twenty-six days in 1988. General hospitals were the major source of admissions (70 percent), and they were the most commonly reported destination for residents discharged alive from LTC facilities. At the end of the decade, hospitals were operating more LTC units (57 units in 1988) than in 1980.

Public Health Care

In August 1989, Governor James Thompson, Cook County Board President George Dunne, and Mayor Richard M. Daley convened the Chicago and Cook County health care summit composed of professional, civic, corporate, and community leaders. The Summit was structured around a policy steering committee of forty-three appointees and a systems design and management committee made up of five subcommittees. The overall purpose was to formulate a series of policy suggestions that the three elected chief executives—two lame ducks—would then be able to take to Springfield for legislative action. As it turned out, the summit recommendations were directed more toward requesting a state funding bailout than toward the initiation of overdue structural reforms within their own bureaucracies by the local chief executives.

The summit schedule was hectic. In its early days, public expectations for reform seemed to grow as a result of the summit's designed process for community input. Nine public hearings across the county drove home the point that public sector health care in Cook County was backward, uncoordinated, and unresponsive. More than 200 people delivered testimony and over 100 submitted written comments. Policymakers noted a clear widespread public dissatisfaction with local health services.

The entire system of care for the poor in Cook County, as well as in the city, had gradually fallen into disarray. For the summit members, as well as those testifying at the summit hearings, there was a consensus that a lack of leadership, vision, and political will in government permitted this deterioration to occur. News coverage of specific health issues had warned political leaders of the growing popular discontent. Reporters and editorial writers of the *Chicago Tribune, Chicago Sun Times*, and *Crain's Chicago Business* addressed health subjects extensively and with increasing frequency over the decade.

The summit did not lead to policy changes or programmatic thrusts, and access to quality primary care today remains critical for the estimated 1.6 million residents of the county who are either uninsured, underinsured, or publicly insured. The public providers—the Chicago Department of Health, Cook County Hospital, Oak Forest Hospital, the Cook County Department of Public Health, and the University of Illinois Hospital and Clinics—have all encountered financial constraints. All distinguished themselves over the decade with increasing levels of mediocrity in their performance. Private hospitals placed barriers to admission for growing numbers of uninsured persons and certain Medicaid recipients. Studies of the practice of "dumping" by private hospitals were conducted at Cook County Hospital, indicating how overburdened this single facility mandated to serve the poor and indigent had become.

County Government

The county government has statutory responsibility for care to the indigent. In Cook County, it operates Cook County Hospital on the Westside of Chicago, Cermak Hospital for prisoners, Oak Forest Hospital in the far south suburbs (mostly for long term care), and the Cook County Department of Public Health. Property tax levies fund the bulk of the expenses for these facilities, as the county has not aggressively pursued increased state and federal reimbursement. Nor has county government sought outside support for medical programs (e.g., foundation grants, philanthropy, or substantial direct patient payments). A new information system designed to facilitate patient billing in Cook County Hospital remains inoperable.

Former Cook County Board President George Dunne obtained a 30 percent spending increase to $1.6 billion for 1990. The county jail and criminal justice system take the lion's share of this budget. Construction of a 1,600-bed correctional facility, which would be a third addition to the county jail—on top of ongoing construction plans for a 1,068-bed jail by 1992—was approved by the County Board in 1990 to alleviate the federally fined overcrowding. The tax rate for health funding actually decreased in 1990, whereas total county health spending increased because of increments in Medicare and Medicaid reimbursements and in property tax collections. About 25 percent of county funds go to health. Increasing county outlays for nonhealth functions may constrain future health capital expenditures, such as the construction of a new county hospital, the renovation of Provident Hospital, or the construction of ambulatory clinics.

Cook County Hospital is notorious for its gross inefficiency. For example, there were about 6,500 employees calculated into its FY 1990 budget of $310 million, which was for a hospital operating at an average daily census (ADC) of 600–650 patients and an annual total of 650,000 outpatient visits (with expenses for its ambulatory-care programs projected to be $37 million). The figures work out to around nine full time equivalent (FTE) employees per adjusted patient day, against a national average for large public hospitals of approximately 5.35. (In contrast, Parkland Memorial Hospital in Dallas has a smaller budget, employs 4,600 workers, but services an ADC of 800 patients, or nearly 200 extra beds.) Over 700,000 ambulatory and emergency room visits flow through Cook County Hospital and its clinics each year, a number that did not increase much over the decade. Because of the hospital's location on the Near Westside of Chicago, it serves the large concentration of poor from the Westside; however, geographic access is problematic for people from the South Side and problems are even greater for the south suburban indigent who must travel over forty miles to receive care.

In October 1987, the Cook County Board of Commissioners decided, after repeated facility postmortems, to move forward in rebuilding the ailing Cook County Hospital. The replacement facility was planned to contain between 696 and 866 beds. At that time, estimated costs of $573.5 million (up to $1.5 billion, including financing costs) were presented to the county board.

Financial constraints amid complicating community politics led to a reconsideration of this decision. Criticism from many quarters of the city was voiced about a "hospital-alone" solution to the mounting uninsured and underserved health problem. Community pressure urged the board to respond to broader health needs among the medically indigent, that is, through better ambulatory-care systems, a strong affiliation between Cook County Hospital and the University of Illinois Hospital, and the purchase of the closed Provident Medical Center. Various groups independent of county government provided policy analyses designed to establish a decentralized, coordinated system of public health care across the county. Intergovernmental cooperation, rather than jurisdictional squabbling, was advocated as a substitute for large new edifices.

The Cook County Board spent well over $100 million dollars during the 1980s in capital renovations for this crumbling hospital. However, in 1990 the Joint Commission on Accreditation of Healthcare Organizations (JCAHO) demanded that another $135 million be spent to meet accreditation standards. For several years, the County Hospital administration had said, in response to JCAHO fire and safety code requirements, that the county board was considering a new facility. Under national scrutiny to tighten its regulatory role, the JCAHO lost patience and demanded that thirty bed wards be eliminated through conversion to semiprivate rooms. Modernization of patient care areas at Cook County has historically been neglected, and renovation schedules have frequently run years behind. The JCAHO finally disaccredited the hospital in April 1990, at the same time that the Health Care Financing Administration (HCFA) was reviewing it for possible withdrawal of its $110 million in Medicare and Medicaid funds. In 1991, HCFA disallowed $20.3 million because of improper outpatient billing.

With regard to quality assurance problems at Cook County Hospital, in 1988 HCFA and the Illinois Department of Public Health threatened to cut off federal and state funds after an inspection found over 200 violations. The inquiries had been provoked by two publicized deaths that had resulted from improper blood transfusions.

Many of the 450 resident physicians at County Hospital are considered by medical observers to fall short of the hospital's past standards of acceptability, even those prevailing at the beginning of the 1980s. Matching has been a major problem for the bulk of the residency programs, most of which are free-standing (i.e., unaffiliated with a medical school) and thus attract mainly foreign medical graduates. Only a few of the hospital's departments have affiliations with the University of Illinois College of Medicine. The surgery affiliation with the University of Illinois was unexpectedly terminated in mid-1990 by the hospital administration. Four residency programs, including general internal medicine, have been on probation; orthopedics was disaccredited; and others were expected to follow the JCAHO disaccreditation.

In the past, the trauma, burn, and neonatal intensive care units of the hospital were known for their exemplary performance, but the current, severe nursing shortage at County Hospital is compromising their standards. Some of the existing medical and nursing staffs of the institution remain dedicated. Overall working conditions have deteriorated however, and no improvements have been made in management systems. Although the medical staff bylaws explicitly prohibit outside private practice, quite a few physicians reportedly work elsewhere on County Hospital time.

The new Cook County Hospital administration appointed by Richard Phelan, the newly elected president of the Cook County Board of Commissioners, faces overwhelming odds: Not only does it have to deal with internal problems accumulated and unaddressed over decades, but it must also address the external, generally uncontrollable, threats from JCAHO, HCFA, and the professional organizations. Phelan's lack of support from the Board of Commissioners further limits his options. It remains to be seen whether significant reform will come quickly or whether initiatives will be instigated only through looming catastrophic episodes in the near future. A growing segment of the Chicago health community expects there to be an inevitable "meltdown" at County Hospital before Provident can be renovated and opened to receive patients in October 1992.

Public awareness and expectations for policy action were raised by the Health Care summit process. Even though no legislative response came out of the recommendations to the state capital in Springfield, the summit focused attention on what needs to be addressed for governmental action. The retirement of County Board President George Dunne and the reelection of Mayor Richard Daley put in place different players for a possible local public health strategy.

A similar opportunity for change occurred when James Thompson ended his fourteen years as governor in 1991. The lame-duck status of Dunne and Thompson—considered two political fossils undistinguished in health policy—and Daley's caution because of reelection fears in April 1991 may have been partially responsible for the postponed implementation of all of the summit suggestions. Other observers have commented on the lack of priority given to health matters by the legislature, particularly in an election year and the presence of a budget crunch with tax implications. Partisan politics rules at the state level in the midst of the real fiscal crisis of the 1990s.

Health Budgets

Public health budgets for the Cook County area increased over the decade. However, the increase was not commensurate with the growing health needs of an at-risk population of 1.6 million with incomes below 200 percent of the poverty level. For FY 1989, the Chicago Department of Health budget was $80.4 million; the amount of city corporate dollars allotted to the department was not much greater than in 1980 because about half of CDOH funds have been federal and state pass-throughs. The county government allocated $181.3 million to Cook County Hospital and $34.8 million to Oak Forest Hospital in FY 1988; these amounts rose considerably during the 1980s as a result of Medicare and Medicaid reimbursements not being aggressively pursued. The Cook County Department of Public Health has a minor budget, which did not grow much over the decade. Total county health appropriations in FY 1989 were $410 million. The state of Illinois has pumped into the University of Illinois Hospital and Clinics a direct subsidy averaging over $10 million a year; in 1988 it was $16.3 million and increased to over $41.5 million in 1989. State Medicaid monies to all Cook County providers were $1.2 billion in FY 1989. The State Department of Health spent an estimated $85 million in grants in Cook County in 1989, up considerably in percent from the beginning of the decade. Total expenditures for health care by all government entities in FY 1989 came to $1.8 billion.

Public Health and Access to Care

Mortality rates for all the leading causes of death in Chicago and Cook County are—as would be expected—significantly higher for nonwhites than for whites, especially in the city. Life expectancy in Chicago (70.4 years vs. 74.7 years for the state) lagged behind the nation as a whole for 1985.

Infant mortality remains a significant problem. The state's overall infant mortality rate was estimated to be 11.6 per 1,000 in 1986, down from 14.7 in 1980. Yet in 1986 the twenty-year-long decline in the infant mortality rate began to reverse. Only eight other states (all southern) had higher rates in 1984. The state government's program target of "9 by 90" is never mentioned anymore in the face of such poor achievement, which is kept low by downstate deaths as well as by continuing problems in Chicago.

The city had an infant mortality rate of 16. 5 per 1,000 in 1986 (then the second highest rate in the nation), 16.6 in 1987, and 15.2 in 1988. In 1986, the rate for blacks, 23 per 1,000, was the highest in the nation, although in subsequent years it was surpassed by the rate in Washington, D.C. Chicago's overall infant mortality rate is now third or fourth highest in the nation. Its 1988 estimate for blacks was 21.4 per 1,000 births; the estimate for Hispanics, particularly Puerto Ricans, remained much lower than that of blacks. Today more than a dozen city neighborhoods have rates in excess of 22, with a few thought to be near 30. By way of contrast, the overall suburban Cook County rate in 1988 was 9.9 per 1,000.

The Social Epidemics

Rising disease rates among the poor and the minority populations of Chicago impose notably greater pressures on public health resources. As throughout the country, but of greater dimension in Chicago, the major disease threats to nonwhites are heart disease, cancer, stroke, trauma, and conditions leading to infant mortality. Accidents, suicide, and especially homicide have distinctively high rates. Unintentional injury rates are higher for the urban poor and working class than for other population groups, particularly in Chicago. The suicide rate for the state rose to 11.1 per 100,000 in 1985, the highest rate since 1950. Young black males in Chicago are more likely to die violent deaths than are black males in other areas. In fact, the city's homicide toll was twice the nation's in 1989, increasing 12 percent in that year alone mostly due to guns. The figures for 1990 and 1991 have even outpaced the 1989 rates. Cancer deaths were up from 188.0 per 100,000 in 1980 to 199.1 in 1985. Following a natural trend, deaths due to heart disease decreased in Illinois where the rate dropped to 349.4 in 1985.

In Chicago, deepening inequalities for blacks are reflected in lower life expectancy and premature loss of life from heart disease, stroke, diabetes, obstructive lung disease, lung cancer, breast cancer, cervical cancer, colorectal cancer, and cirrhosis of the liver. The higher mortality among blacks is due not only to higher disease rates than among whites but also to delayed detection and inadequate treatment. It should be noted that these chronic conditions are all to some extent preventable by reducing risk factors, including cigarette smoking, obesity, high blood pressure, alcohol consumption, lack of exercise, and hazardous occupational conditions. Lack of information on signs and symptoms; economic, social, and cultural barriers to adequate primary care and preventive services; and improper medical follow-up account in part for the higher death rates among blacks, especially among poor and working-class people. Higher death and disease rates due to infection, and a much greater severity of illness, are noted among the lower classes, as witnessed in the 1988-1989 measles and influenza epidemics, which rocked Chicago's public health care services.

AIDS is spreading rapidly within Chicago's black and Hispanic communities, although the city's rate is relatively low compared to several other large cities. However, the AIDS Foundation of Chicago estimated a 39 percent increase in the total number of AIDS cases for 1990, compared to a 4 percent increase in 1988. There were 1,153 new cases reported in Illinois in 1989, an increase of 16 percent over 1988. Since IDPH began collecting data on AIDS in 1981, 3,509 cases have been reported throughout the state, 2,552 of them in Chicago. Seventy-two percent of adult cases are homosexual or bisexual males. As elsewhere, AIDS now afflicts minorities and women to a much greater extent than previously reported. Chicago health officials in 1989 commented on the problem of underreporting in their *AIDS Strategic Plan.* A 1989 profile of Chicago intravenous (IV) drug users found 19.1 percent of North Side and 15.6 percent of South Side IV drug users testing positive for HIV.

State attention to AIDS has been anything but impressive. For Illinois, total state spending in FY 1989 was $5.6 million, placing it seventh when compared to other states. The state's 1989 AIDS spending came to a mere forty-nine cents per capita. (By comparison, California, the highest ranking state, spent $76 million, and the District of Columbia spent $9.91 per capita.) Earlier last decade a number of restrictive legislative bills were introduced in Springfield. One of them, which required AIDS testing before marriage, was passed, driving couples out of state. Hardly any cases of AIDS among newly married couples were detected during the lifetime of the law, and it was rescinded in 1989. The city government faced a rocky road in implementing its AIDS program until its *AIDS Strategic Plan,* adopted in October 1989, intensified efforts to involve a broader community in order to build consensus on funding allocations.

Sexually transmitted diseases were particularly problematic at the end of the decade. As elsewhere, rates for gonorrhea climbed dramatically, but syphilis continued to go undetected and untreated. Despite assistance by the U.S. Centers for Disease Control, the Cook County Department of Public Health has failed miserably in stemming the growing numbers, especially in the southern suburbs. The Chicago Department of Health reportedly has improved its delivery of services for STDs in the face of the rising epidemics.

Substance abuse is also on the rise, especially in the city. Crack came to Chicago late, in 1988. For reasons that are unclear, Chicago gangs held off on major distribution of this form of cocaine, but its seizure rate exploded on the South Side and in the suburbs starting in 1989. Neonatal intensive care units report growing numbers of babies afflicted with traces of drugs and full addictions, and growing numbers of drug-caused infant deaths.

Drugs have severely complicated the low-birth-weight problems of babies born to black teens.

Insurance Coverage

In Chicago, the problem of medical indigency intensified severely during the 1980s. The Chicago Health Systems Agency estimated in 1986 that 20 percent of the population was chronically uninsured. This guesstimate was based on an extrapolation of data from the 1977 National Medical Care Expenditures Survey and was not properly adjusted for the effects of federal health cutbacks, the ongoing decline in midwestern manufacturing, or the rapid growth of the service industries in the area. Over 21 percent of Chicagoans are covered by Medicaid, and now over 12 percent are on Medicare. Thus, the ranks of the poor and the indigent exceed 1.6 million; the number is even higher when one adds those whose private health insurance (or Medicare) is insufficient to pay for their medical expenses.

Blue Cross/Blue Shield of Illinois is estimated to have a market share of less than 18 percent, an amount that declined over the decade. Other private health insurance, employer self-insurance, and PPOs constitute approximately 30 percent of the market. HMOs have a 12 percent market share today, which includes about 130,000 Medicaid beneficiaries who enrolled since the Illinois Department of Public Aid began contracting in March 1984. (Note that figures for these categories are not mutually exclusive.)

Trends in the hospital sector indicate a worsening financial picture in general, but there is a disturbing variability among hospitals. A major problem exists in the indicators used to spell out the real danger. It should not be concluded that the poor outlook is due solely to government underfunding and to the response the hospitals have been forced to make to the indigence burden. In their defense, Chicago area hospitals received only 11 percent of their total revenues in 1986 from the Medicaid program for 15 percent of their days, indicating restricted payments as well as eligibility. The disproportionate share funding in 1989 by the legislature eased the relative burden on certain inner-city hospitals.

The hospital industry calculated an "uncompensated-care" expense for the metropolitan area of over $400 million for 1986; this number has remained flat over the subsequent years. (In 1984, the estimated figure was $434 million for the entire state.) Three quarters of the $400 million expense has been linked to care provided by hospitals in the city. The Metropolitan Chicago Healthcare Council calculates this expense to amount to 8 percent of gross patient service revenues. For hospitals in Cook County, the bulk of the uncompensated care was delivered by the two public institutions (one-third by Cook County Hospital and the University of Illinois Hospital, the latter before its change of mission) and three major teaching hospitals (Michael Reese before the Humana takeover, Mount Sinai, and the University of Chicago). As elsewhere, the most expensive institutions tend to take care of the neediest patients, though ICARE has succeeded in redirecting some of the Medicaid patient flow.

Unfortunately, there has been little honest attempt by the hospital associations to analyze the trend in uncompensated care to delineate its true components. The figure is based on unpaid bills from charge data, not actual costs, so in reality it is not a measure of unsponsored patient losses, let alone the often cited charity care. Write-offs of all sorts from Medicare and Medicaid, adjustments to private patient charges, bad debts, and the like are often included in the figure, which inflates the determination of the actual loss the local hospitals must bear for lack of universal coverage for all Illinois residents.

The two hospital groups, the Metropolitan Chicago Health Care Council and the Illinois Hospital Association unfortunately, have a trade-association mentality, according to outside observers. Even the proposal of mandated benefits for the uninsured by the Illinois Hospital Association, known as ACT (Accessible Care Today), was viewed as sad evidence of self-interest because it urged mainly inpatient coverage.

Much anecdotal evidence is offered about the sizable increases in the use of emergency rooms by uninsured patients, but these increases may be attributable to the fact that only patients who have been admitted are potentially eligible to be "MANGed, " that is to be classified for reimbursement by the state as "Medical Assistance, No Grant." This mechanism in Illinois permits near-impoverished hospitalized patients who face extraordinary hospital bills to be enrolled in Medicaid. For 1988, MANG expenditures in Cook County for inpatient care were $153 million. A 1989 Medicaid change allowed MANG and AMI ("Aid to Medically Indigent") recipients to receive benefits if their medical costs exceeded their assets and income.

Notwithstanding this effort to recover some losses, all hospitals appear to be relying upon collection firms to extract some payment from their non-full pay patients, though their first tactic has been to try to transfer these patients to public sector hospitals. However, according to the ER medical administrator at Cook County Hospital, "dumping" of patients onto the public sector has not continued at the alarming rate seen in the mid-1980s.

Many uninsured, as well as underinsured, patients pay out-of-pocket for primary care provided by their "local medical doctors" and also for emergency room visits; the uninsured and underinsured use a smaller volume of hospital services than do the well insured. Their lower admissions rate probably reflects their younger age profile; however, lower utilization may reflect increased barriers to care, even in the overcrowded public sector. Nevertheless, it is generally believed that if one is really in need of hospitalization, it can be had in the Chicago area; it is in primary care and follow-up care that huge numbers of people are denied necessary and timely services.

Medicaid patients are reportedly sicker than other patient groups when hospitalized. Some physicians claim these patients must be very sick to be admitted, saying that hospitals are frequently reluctant to accept them given the inadequate payment by the state. In the past couple of years, hospitals did not use all of their contracted ICARE days as they previously had. Apparently, temporary adjustments in hospital behavior occurred, and the state achieved a "savings" of nearly $400 million over the years 1985–1989 from ICARE. This program has apparently realized one of its early goals, that of shifting some care to the less expensive institutions. Nevertheless, IDPA incurred a budget shortfall of over $300 million for Medicaid in FY 1991, and the new governor, Jim Edgar, requested only an additional $185 million in his first budget for the program. That amount did not cover the deficit, let alone the expected inflation in Medicaid. In the spring of 1991, the state owed over $600 million in back bills for social and medical programs, with payment delays of nearly ninety days. In Edgar's FY 1992 budget, $570 million have been cut from other health and human services, which will, no doubt, eliminate much of the "safety net" that prevents or postpones the more costly hospital interventions.

One might speculate that the community populations have altered their behavior as well. The message gets out quickly that Medicaid and indigent patients are unwanted at certain hospitals and that other institutions, at which Medicaid recipients account for more than 50 percent of their patient days, are the places to go. Some private hospitals have eliminated, downsized, or closed their outpatient departments to new entrants. Fire department and private ambulance teams learn to seek the "proper" base hospital in the EMS system. Whether their doing so is a subtle form of economic triage is uncertain, although studies in other cities have found evidence of similar situations. When locational choices are present, more obvious changes in patient flows may be complementing the intended ICARE repatterning of patient distribution (to lower cost hospitals). This problem awaits empirical investigation. The disaccredited Cook County Hospital remains the only provider of last resort for the county population.

Beyond these observations and speculations, other changes in utilization patterns for the indigent are difficult to ascertain. Operating statistics reveal a general stabilizing of ambulatory visits at both Fantus Clinic of Cook County Hospital and the Chicago Department of Health clinics over the past few years. The CDOH clinics record about 1 million encounters annually, counting each incident of service. CCH ambulatory-care totals remain at about 750,000 for ER, ambulatory screening, and scheduled outpatient visits. The University of Illinois clinics had 350,000 visits, though this number has declined somewhat following the change in the University of Illinois Hospital's mission statement. No big jumps in outpatient volumes elsewhere have been noticeable.

Whether people are just "doing without" remains a question; it is known that small private group practices (not all of them Medicaid mills) serve a large number of inner-city neighborhoods. Because poor and indigent residents receive little or no routine care, many practitioners feel that a higher incidence of childhood illnesses, lower rates of immunization, and the like may empirically show up later in disease statistics. However, surveillance mechanisms for such matters are not really in place in Chicago; neither are targeted health planning strategies, except in the area of infant mortality, and these have not been deemed effective. There is no exchange of data sets, let alone much coordination of effort, among the public providers, though an assessment of these issues did come out of the Chicago and Cook County Health Care Summit.

Possibilities for Coordination

The Chicago and Cook County Health Care Summit recognized the contribution of the community-based neighborhood health centers, some of which were continuing to operate under federal 330 funding. Although a few centers grew in volume over the decade (and a couple of small ones were launched), there were coincident service cutbacks at several due to financial problems. The closure of the Miles Square Health Center on the Westside after several years of spiraling down, left a huge gap. It has since been reopened by the University of Illinois in collaboration with the Chicago Department of Health. This former federally funded but community-controlled 330-bed facility, which had been the largest community-based health program for the poor on the Westside, was shuttered for over two years.

Including the CDOH- and Cook County Hospital-sponsored sites, Chicago has fifty-eight neighborhood clinics, which could potentially be brought together in an organized system of ambulatory care for the county. With public provider assistance (clinical and managerial) and greater government funding, these private not-for-profit ambulatory ventures (and others to be created in the summit's designated "corridors" of neighborhood need) could supplement the overcrowded public facilities and extend access significantly. Linkage agreements for referral mechanisms, computerized records and billing, and ancillary services backup have been discussed. The summit process was intended to speed up such actions, but relatively little by way of outcomes has resulted.

An attempt is under way to capture more federal dollars through Medicaid by creating a local fund. Initially a proposal of the Health and Medicine Policy Research Group, this pooling of state, county, and city expenditures for the medically indigent follows the efforts of other states to tally a greater amount of indigent care in order to increase the federal contribution to Medicaid. It is estimated that up to $200 million in new federal monies could be added to pay for care for the indigent in Illinois. Capturing these federal dollars would necessitate converting $315 million of city, county, and state funds already allocated for medical care delivery to state funds. The legality of such a strategy (will the Health Care Financing Administration grant a waiver?) and the willingness of city and county Democrats to turn over funds to a Republican state administration remain problematic. The state legislature has refused to consider it in two sessions so far.

The demand for ambulatory care in Cook County is estimated to exceed current capacity by over 2 million visits annually. Barriers to care, over and above a lack of insurance coverage, are numerous, ranging from cultural insensitivity to lack of child care and transportation. A significant number of current users of public sector facilities are Medicaid-eligible but not enrolled. The Health Care Summit calculated that over $32 million in Medicaid monies could be captured by Cook County Hospital and the Chicago Department of Health clinics if those who were currently eligible were enrolled.

Proposals for the integration of public health care services have included strengthening the role of the University of Illinois Health Sciences Center. As a step in this direction, a medical clinic with broad nursing and clinical pharmacy functions was established in 1990 by the University at the old St. Anne's Hospital Professional Office Building in the Austin community. The university-city collaboration at Miles Square Health Center in 1991 shows additional commitment, though its board of trustees offered considerable political resistance to the reopening. The significance of these and a few other faculty initiatives lies not simply in the new (though limited) university outreach they represent but also in the intergovernmental cooperation they elicited.

Over time, the quality of care in the city and county health facilities has been compromised by too many patients, a lack of satisfactory equipment and qualified and motivated staff, inadequate physical plants, and so forth. Early joint efforts to improve the university–Cook County Hospital relationship portend brighter prospects. Health services research, along with clinical research, may aid in the development of innovative, effective programs as models of coordination for the public and private sectors.

Clearly, access to health care has been defined as a major problem in the Cook County area. Media attention, from the daily newspapers to *Crain's*

Chicago Business and the *Chicago Reporter*, was reflected in a few public information series as well as in lengthy coverage of policy reports and summit developments. Broad community support for action was noted in the public hearings of the summit. It is generally felt that community-based programs have been better received by the public and are more effective than those externally mounted and operated. The timing and the extent of any new governmental response by way of coordination, backup, and increased funding will determine whether there will be any significant change in the future. However, the provision of new political leadership for health by Governor Edgar, Richard Phelan (the Cook County Board president), or Mayor Daley remains doubtful at this time.

Public Policy

The issue of access to care dominated policy discussions of the 1980s in Illinois, but little more than tinkering actually was done by the state government. In 1988-1989, a Governor's Health Care Summit (involving the Departments of Public Health and Public Aid, the Health Care Facilities Planning Board, the Health Care Cost Containment Council, and the Health Facilities Authority) devised a new "policy agenda." The summit was a timely event, somewhat forced by the widespread perception (and the reality) that state government was grossly ineffective in responding to a growing set of health needs statewide—not just in Chicago. However, as was the case over the decade, the main obstacles to adoption and implementation of suggested actions became the lack of money and the failure to exercise political will—by the former governor, his agencies, and the Democratic majority of the legislature.

With regard to health care in Illinois, the 1980s can best be described as a decade of postponement, with small incremental state funding for new health programs and ineffective measures for cost control over Medicaid. Policymakers studied health issues and wrote reports ad infinitum, but the reports failed to alter priorities in Governor Thompson's administration. One example of decisive action taken was the legislature's embarrassing mandate for AIDS testing prior to the issuance of a marriage license; it caused couples to cross the state borders to get married, cost over $2 million to implement, and led to the detection of only eight AIDS cases.

The pattern of commissions, summits, conferences, and studies but no courageous system restructuring was reflected in Chicago and Cook County as well. As discussed earlier, the 1990 state legislature adjourned without taking action on any of the Chicago and Cook County Health Care Summit recommendations. Neither the proposal for a Cook County Health Council to coordinate public sector care nor the stronger model of a Regional Health Authority proposed by the Health and Medicine Policy

Research Group received attention. The suggestion of pooling city and county local funds into Medicaid to try to capture greater federal financing was likewise ignored. Thus, Illinois still has not confronted its growing problem of citizens who are uninsured or underinsured for health care. The limited capacity of the governments of Cook County and the city of Chicago to provide expanded, more effective services to low income residents intensifies the crisis.

Plagued by rampant inflation in overall costs, the Medicaid program in Illinois expanded benefits little in the 1980s except where forced to do so by federal mandate. Although the state took advantage of a Health Care Financing Administration waiver for the ICARE program to provide for competitive bidding, Illinois has moved grudgingly on maternal-child health and other improvements. Along with perpetual, bitter conflicts with the hospitals, the Illinois Department of Public Aid experienced chronic shortfalls in its available funds. For several years, it ran out of money before the end of the fiscal year, requiring new, last-minute appropriations by the state legislature after payment delays of up to four months. The Illinois Hospital Association requested that claims be paid within thirty days and that more coverage be granted for women and children (as federal law permits). They also want increases in ambulatory services and physician payments (raised in 1989 to $18 per doctor visit for most hospitals, although a few institutional rates were granted to community health centers and CDOH clinics) as well as larger payments for trauma, burn, and other specialty services. Historically, any increases in the Medicaid budget have come only after funding for public schools, higher education, correctional facility construction and modernization, and the removal of mental patients from nursing homes as per federal order have been addressed.

Beyond the decreased demand for services, the major complaint of city-based hospitals focuses on Medicaid reimbursement. For example, in 1988 for the thirteen Westside hospitals, four of which are teaching institutions, the ICARE program supposedly paid "costs" ranging from 60 percent to percentages in the mid-30s. The governor's 1988 budget proposed a small inflationary increase, and the state legislature waited another year before enacting a "temporary" income tax in response to loud public clamor for increased spending for education. AFDC payments under welfare were also increased slightly, the first such increase in over a decade. Given this situation, coupled with Medicare DRG restrictions (about which not much complaint is heard from the hospitals) and other prospective payments, it is estimated that perhaps 50 percent of the city's hospitals had negative operating margins in the latter years of the 1980s. On a more positive note, the state's fair-share grants to hospitals in 1989 alleviated the plight of certain institutions whose patient mix included 25 percent or more Medicaid clients by increasing Medicaid per diem rates between $40 and $230 for forty-six institutions.

Like Medicaid reform, the Accessible Health Care Act, the Illinois Hospital Association's proposal to provide coverage for the growing numbers of uninsured, has not gotten on the public agenda. Not known as an advocate for the poor, the IHA sought mandated insurance benefits for all workers. For this to pass, the vested interests of the IHA and the Illinois State Medical Society would have to unite (an infrequent occurrence) and take on the Chamber of Commerce, which is composed of all the small businesses. The large Illinois corporations are not showing much interest in state health care initiatives, though a move is afoot in Chicago to bring business groups together under the Chicago Partnership to examine health care, as they did in the case of school reform. Cynics remark that the health care system is far more complex than education and in more desperate need of complete restructuring, which entails greater political risks and requires greater sophistication than the passage of a single piece of "reform" legislation.

A beginning progressive constituency of professionals, consumer and religious groups, and some provider agencies contends that far-reaching public policy solutions are now necessary in the city and throughout the state. Activism for universal health insurance has appeared in the form of newsletters, conferences, and draft legislation but is not as vigorous as in California and a few other states. A coalition of organizations, which formed the Campaign for Better Health Care, enticed Representative Marty Russo to aid its state legislative efforts. A long-time Democrat from south Chicago and the Cook County suburbs, Russo submitted a Canadian-style national health insurance bill to Congress in 1991.

On the whole, Chicago's health delivery system has been laggard when compared to many other metropolitan regions where private and public provider restructuring and progressive state health initiatives moved forward more rapidly over the 1980s. Whether considering the degree of multi-institutional provider development, proprietarization, out-of-hospital amalgamation, or interorganizational linkages, Chicago as an area has not been in the forefront, as indicated in the health and hospital trade magazines. Although the Cook County and Chicago public health care sector can be uniquely characterized as the most backward, the private health sector also failed to participate in certain trends until recently in the way that the academic and religious multi-institutional providers did. The few glimmers that began in 1988 indicate a turning point among the voluntary providers. Unfortunately, the strategy of private corporate expansion will not resolve the mounting public health and indigent care problems.

In summary, developments that were generally *not* expected in Chicago when looking forward from the year 1980 were (1) the large number of hospital closures in the city; (2) the intensification of the issue of long-term care in terms of objective needs and nursing home utilization; (3) the expanding AIDS epidemic, as well as the resurgence of infectious disease entities like TB; (4) the nursing shortage; and (5) Medicaid underfunding relative to the growing numbers of uninsured persons in the state. Given the degree of competition in the health care sector in metropolitan Chicago, interviewees often remarked how surprised they were that the HMO market had not grown more than it did. Although most observers had expected the regulatory-planning approach to fall out of favor, others noted that gross inefficiencies had not been eliminated from the system. Pessimism concerning the public sector—state, county, and city—remains widespread and is deepening, although more insiders today are recognizing that a stronger government role must be forthcoming at least on the access issue. Because of significant activism and media attention, policymakers today have greater in-depth knowledge of health and health care system problems. So does the public.

For Illinois, the state and local roles in health policy formulation are more crucial than what has transpired at the national level. Despite its powerful politicians in Congress, Illinois has lagged sorely in per capita federal spending, ranking forty-sixth among the states in 1989. Federal health and human services spending amounted to $2,176 million in grants and $4,968 million in Medicaid monies; the low ranking came from the lack of defense spending. More important for a reform agenda, the design and operations of the metropolitan Chicago health care system seem to be shaped mainly by the historical political culture of the state and the locale. The mounting local needs and the system's failings have become driving forces for change; what is now necessary is a more unified, consistent, and powerful constituency to force the political will toward overdue structural reform and greater targeted funding.

Bibliography

Abraham, L., "Dallas Public Hospital: A Lesson for County?" *Chicago Reporter* 19 (1990): 3–11.

———. "Jumble of Health Rules Limits Care for Poor," *Chicago Reporter* 18 (1989): 3–5.

American Hospital Association, *Hospital Statistics, 1987* (Chicago: American Hospital Association, 1987).

Berkeley, L., Salmon, J.W. et al., *Towards Better Health for Chicago: Challenges and Opportunities. Report of the Needs Assessment Committee for Health/Disability* (Chicago: United Way of Chicago, 1990).

Better Business Association, *A Consumer Guide to Long Term Care Facilities, Cook County, Illinois* (Chicago: Better Business Administration, 1990).

Chicago Department of Health, *AIDS Strategic Plan* (Chicago: Department of Health, 1989).

———. *An Approach to Financing Level I Trauma Care* (Chicago: Department of Health, 1989).

———. *Clinics in Crisis: A Report on the Conditions and Capacity of the Chicago Department of Health's Clinic Facilities* (Chicago: Department of Health, 1989).

———. *City of Chicago Community Area Health Inventory* (Chicago: Department of Health, 1986).

Chicago Health Executives Forum, "Healthcare: Business or Public Service? An Analysis of the Mission and Financial Commitment of Chicago-Area Hospitals to Public Service" (Chicago: Chicago Health Executives Forum, January 12, 1990).

Chicago Health Systems Agency, *Health Systems Plan* (Chicago: Chicago Health Systems Agency, 1987).

Chicago Hospital Council, *Facts About Hospitals in Metropolitan Chicago, 1990* (Chicago: Chicago Hospital Council, 1990).

Chicago Tribune, "Ignoring the Public Health Disaster," June 17, 1990, Sec. 1.

Crain's Chicago Business, "Humana Seeks Reese at Discount," October 25, 1990, 1.

Fossett, J.W., Peterson, J.A., Ring, M.C., *The Invisible Providers: Public Sector Primary Care and Medicaid* (Chicago: University of Illinois at Chicago Institute for Government and Public Affairs, 1988).

Griffith, J.L., "In Grave Condition: Latest Attempt to Rescue Health System Falling Short," *Chicago Tribune*, June 11, 1990, 1, 10.

———. "Plan Seeks to Revamp County Health Care," *Chicago* Tribune, April 1, 1990, 1.

Illinois Department of Public Aid, *Avenues Toward Self Sufficiency: Long Term Care* (Springfield, IL: Illinois Department of Public Aid, 1989).

———. *Avenues Toward Self Sufficiency: Medical Assistance Programs* (Springfield, IL: Illinois Department of Public Aid, 1989).

———. *Meeting the Challenge: Growth and Progress* (Springfield: Illinois Department of Public Aid, 1986).

Illinois Department of Public Health, *Report on Long Term Care Facilities Illinois—* 1987-88 (Springfield, IL: Illinois Department of Public Health, 1989).

———. 1988 Human Services Plan, Part 1 Data Report (Springfield, IL: Illinois Department of Public Health, 1988).

———. *Proprietary Health Care Facilities and Services in Illinois* (Springfield, IL: Illinois Department of Public Health, Office of Health Policy and Planning, Division of Health Information and Evaluation, 1988).

Illinois Health Care Cost Containment Council, *The Evolution of National Health Policy and the Illinois Health Care Delivery System* (Springfield, IL: Illinois Health Care Cost Containment Council, 1986).

Illinois Hospital Association, Center for Health Affairs, *Illinois Hospitals Quarterly Financial Condition Report:* 12 Months Ending June 30, 1986 (Naperville, IL: Illinois Hospital Association, 1986).

_____ . Task Force on Indigent Care, *Financing of Health Care for the Medically Indigent in a Common Marketplace* (Naperville, IL: Illinois Hospital Association, 1986).

Institute of Medicine of Chicago, *Health Care for the Inner City of Chicago: Conference Report*. (Chicago: Institute of Medicine, 1983).

Marsh, B., "The Medical Indigence Crisis: Chicago's Working Poor Fall Into Widening Insurance Gap," *Crain's Chicago Business* 11(43), October 24–30, 1988.

_____ . "Sleepy Catholic Hospitals' Giant Awakening," *Crain's Chicago Business*, March 21, 1988.

Merrion, P., "Illinois Services Growth Trails National Gain," *Crain's Chicago Business*, January 7, 1990.

Metropolitan Chicago Healthcare Council, *Utilization of Short-term General and Specialty Hospitals in Metropolitan Chicago for the Third Quarter of 1989* (Chicago: Metropolitan Chicago Healthcare Council, 1989).

_____ . *Financial Facts and Trends About Metropolitan Chicago Hospitals* (Chicago: Metropolitan Chicago Healthcare Council, 1989).

_____ . *Elderly Healthcare: Addressing the Need* (Chicago: Metropolitan Chicago Healthcare Council, 1988).

_____ . "Illinois HMOs: An Overview of Today's Market and Future Directions," *HMO/PPO Tracking Report* 4(2), pp. 1, 17–18, 1988.

_____ . "Preferred Provider Organizations: Planning for Growth and Change," *HMO/PPO Tracking Report* 4(4), pp. 1–3, 1988.

_____ . *Public Aid Inpatient Contracting and Its Impact on Hospitals and Recipients* (Chicago: Metropolitan Chicago Healthcare Council, 1988).

_____ . *The Health Care Cost Problem: Toward a Long Term Solution* (Chicago: Metropolitan Chicago Healthcare Council, 1987).

Millenson, M., "Eight Illinois Hospitals Cited for High Death Rates," *Chicago Tribune*, December 21, 1989, Sec. 2, p. 3.

Mitchell, L., Griffith, J.L., "In Grave Condition: Politics Cripples Health-Care Reform," *Chicago Tribune*, June 12, 1990, pp. 1, 18.

Mount, C., "$1.6 Billion County Budget Proposed," *Chicago Tribune*, December 20, 1989, Sec. 2, p. 1.

Nemes, J., "Humana Won't Need CON for Michael Reese," *Modern Healthcare* (November 12, 1990), p. 4.

Oloroso, A., "Health Summit Proposals Hit Political Wall," *Crain's Chicago Business*, May 24, 1990, p. 3.

_____ . "Study: Hospitals Not Earning Tax-Exempt Status," *Crain's Chicago Business*, January 1, 1990, p. 4.

Policy Steering Committee, Chicago and Cook County Health Care Summit, "Statement of Principles," Mimeograph (Chicago: Department of Health, February, 1990).

_____ . "Oral and Written Testimony Synopsis," Mimeograph (Chicago: Department of Health, February, 1990).

Reynolds, G., "Curing Chicago's Hospital Crisis," *Chicago Magazine*, July 1990, pp. 88–91, 114–117.

Salmon, J.W., "Learning from Other Urban Public Healthcare Settings," in Joseph, L. (ed.)., *Paying for Healthcare in Illinois*. (Chicago: University of Chicago Center for Urban Research and Policy Studies. Distributed by University of Illinois Press, 1991).

———— . "Translation into Political Practice: Experience from the Health and Medicine Policy Research Group, Chicago, Illinois" (Prepared for Zukunftsaufgabe Gesundheitsfoerderung Kongress, sponsored by Aertzekammer Berlin; Landesverband der Betriebskrankenkassen, Berlin; Facultaet Soziologie, Technische Universitaet der Berlin; und Regionalbuero fuer Europa, World Health Organization, April 30, 1989).

———— . "The Uninsured and the Underinsured: What Can We Do?" *The Internist: Health Policy in Practice* 29(4) (1988): 8–13.

———— . (ed.), *The Corporate Transformation of Healthcare, Part I: Issues and Directions* (Amityville, NY: Baywood, 1990).

———— . (ed.), *Proceedings of the Health and Medicine Policy Research Group Conference "Towards a Cook County Public Health Care Delivery System, April 25, 1986"* (Chicago: Health and Medicine Policy Research Group, 1987).

Salmon, J.W., Lieber, H.S., Ayesse, M.C., "Reducing Inpatient Hospital Costs: An Attempt at Medicaid Reform in Illinois," *Journal of Health Politics, Policy and Law* 13(1) (1988): 103–127.

Salmon, J.W., Todd, J.W. (eds.), *Proceedings of "The Corporatization of Health Care: A Two Day Symposium and Public Hearing"* (Springfield, IL: Illinois Public Health Association, 1988).

State of Illinois, Bureau of the Budget, *Illinois Population Trends, 1980 to 2025* (Springfield, IL: State of Illinois, Bureau of the Budget, 1987).

———— . Statewide Health Coordinating Council, *Health Needs, Vol.* 1: Illinois Health Needs and Priorities Statement, Part 1 (Springfield, IL: State of Illinois, Office of the Governor, 1981).

Systems Design and Management Committee, *Chicago and Cook County Health Care Action Plan: Report of the Chicago and Cook County Health Care Summit (Volume I: Executive Summary)* (Chicago: Chicago Department of Health, 1990).

———— . *Chicago and Cook County Health Care Summit: Health Care System Overview; Summary of Existing Plans* (Chicago: Chicago Department of Health, 1990).

University of Illinois at Chicago, College of Nursing, *Proceedings of the Seminar "Primary Health Care in Chicago"* (Chicago: University of Illinois, December 1989).

Urban Institute Non-Profit Sector Project, *Hardship and Support Systems in Chicago: A Summary of Recent Findings,* (Chicago: Urban Institute, 1986).

Webber, H., Salmon, J.W. et al., *Foundations for Policy Decisions for a New Cook County Public Health Care Delivery System: Options for Governance* (Chicago: Health and Medicine Policy Research Group, 1988).

Whiteis, D., "The Provider of Last Resort," *Chicago Reader,* April 7, 1989, p. 1.

Whiteis, D., Salmon, J.W., *Public Healthcare Delivery Systems in Selected U.S. Cities: Findings of the Urban Public Health Care Systems Tours Project,* Report to the Field Foundation of Chicago (Chicago: University of Illinois, College of Pharmacy, 1990).

Young, Q., Salmon J.W. et al., *Breaking the Mold: A New Vision for a Cook County Public Health Care Delivery System* (Chicago: Health and Medicine Policy Research Group, 1986).

_____ . *Toward a Cook County Public Health Care System: A New Vision* (Chicago: Health and Medicine Policy Research Group, 1986).

In addition, over forty health policymakers, analysts, and practitioners were interviewed over the three-year course of this Columbia University Eisenhower Center for the Conservation of Human Resources project and newspaper coverage of healthcare issues was followed. I am deeply indebted to each person for the time and information contributed to this monitoring effort. The counsel of colleagues from organizations in which I have participated as a volunteer is also acknowledged with gratitude. Special thanks are due to Maggie Santos, Penelopee D. Bankhead, and Lawana Elliott for their supportive efforts in the preparation of the manuscript.

4

Changing Health Care in Los Angeles:
Poverty Amid Affluence,
Competition Leading to Crisis

E. Richard Brown and Geraldine Dallek

Los Angeles comprises at least two different cities in terms of health care, wealth, housing, education, and other basic elements of health and human life. It is a metropolis in which private care with the most advanced medical technology is readily available to its affluent, well-insured population and is available with some limitations on access to its middle-income insured population that is increasingly enrolled in managed-care plans. At the same time, another Los Angeles provides poor access to limited care for its vast uninsured, largely low-income population. The 1980s were characterized by an increasing divergence of these realities. The first part of this chapter describes the metropolis, its population, and the distribution of power and influence in medicine.

Three trends have caused increasing health care problems for all people in Los Angeles. One problem has been the diversification and decline of health insurance, which has led to increasing frustrations for much of the privately insured population and the rapid growth of an uninsured population that is dependent on the public "safety net." A second problem has been the increasing burdens the public sector has had to bear without adequate financial or political support. Finally, the frantic competition among health care providers for revenues and resources has exacerbated all other problems and threatened the very survival of many health care facilities and services. The chapter concludes with a discussion of the political outlook for solutions to these problems.

Poverty and Wealth in Los Angeles

Population

Los Angeles is the population, economic, political, and cultural center of southern California and of the state. Los Angeles County's more than nine million residents represent about one third of the state's population. The six counties that make up southern California generated $140 billion in goods and services in 1980, 5.3 percent of the U.S. gross national product. Los Angeles is thus an economically important and affluent metropolis.

For more than a century, Los Angeles has been a magnet for migrants from every region of the United States and other countries, and it has retained this attraction in recent years. Between 1980 and 1987, Los Angeles became the home of 387,663 more people than left it, with migration contributing 39 percent of the net population increase in those seven years.

The population of Los Angeles is ethnically diverse, containing large numbers of immigrants from Mexico and the rest of Latin America, from Asia and the Pacific Islands, and from Europe. One quarter of all foreign-born persons in the United States live in California, and almost half of the state's foreign-born population live in Los Angeles. In 1980, 6 percent of the U.S. population was foreign-born, compared to 15 percent in California and 22 percent in Los Angeles. A majority (55 percent) of the foreign-born population in Los Angeles in 1980 came from Latin America; another 13 percent came from Asia, and 20 percent came from Europe. By 1986, 93,300 Southeast Asian refugees had settled in Los Angeles. Estimates of the number of undocumented immigrants range as high as 1.5 million, although the true figure is probably closer to 1 million.

The county is dominated by de facto residential segregation, with ethnic groups concentrated in small pockets and in huge sprawling areas. Mexicans, Central Americans (especially Salvadorans and Guatemalans), Koreans, Japanese, and Chinese all live in large, identifiable communities dominated by immigrant and first-generation members of these groups. Southeast Asians, Pacific Islanders, Armenians, and other newcomer populations occupy smaller pockets, often scattered over wide portions of the county. African-Americans are concentrated in south-central Los Angeles but also live in large numbers elsewhere in the county.

Between 1980 and 1990, non-Latino whites became another minority group, representing 41 percent of the residents of Los Angeles County, although they remain the most affluent and politically and socially dominant segment of the population. The number of Latinos, both American-born and immigrant, rose to three and one-half million, constituting 39 percent of the population. Blacks, Asians, and other racial minorities account for 10 percent each.

The Economy

During the 1970s and 1980s, Los Angeles experienced simultaneous industrial contraction and expansion, which led to job loss in some manufacturing industries and job expansion in others and to the creation of more jobs in the service and retail sectors of the economy. Between 1979 and 1987, the number of manufacturing jobs in Los Angeles declined by 2 percent, from 925,000 to 907,000; in comparison, the number of manufacturing jobs in New York fell 25 percent (to 461,000) and in Chicago, 35 percent (to 551, 000). This relative stability in total manufacturing jobs in Los Angeles masks a shift from the heavily unionized, well-paying durable goods producing sector, in which the number of jobs declined by 3 percent during this period (half the national decline of 6 percent), to the less unionized, often low-wage nondurable goods sector, in which the number of jobs increased by 18 percent (against a drop of 5 percent nationally). During the 1970s and 1980s, retail and service sector jobs grew in Los Angeles as they did throughout the rest of the country; together they accounted for 49 percent of total employment in Los Angeles in 1987, compared to 47 percent nationally.

The economic restructuring has led to a widening gap between the poor and the more affluent. In Los Angeles, the poorest fifth of all families received only 9.8 percent of the income received by the richest fifth in 1987, which was virtually the same as in 1979 (9.7 percent) but well below the percentage in 1969 (11.8 percent). The disparity in Los Angeles is greater than that in the nation as a whole, in which the poorest fifth of families received 10.5 percent of the income received by the richest fifth in 1987, compared to 12.5 percent in 1979 and 13.8 percent in 1969. As these data suggest, a greater percentage of the population in Los Angeles lives below the poverty level (15.6 percent in 1987) than in the United States as a whole (13.5 percent), the reverse of the pattern in 1969.

In 1980, 10 percent of U.S. -born residents in Los Angeles aged sixteen to sixty-four were living in poverty, which was about half the rate for residents born in Central America, South America, or Asia and less than half the rate for those born in Mexico.

Power and Health Care

The changing composition of the population of Los Angeles only recently has been reflected in the political establishment in the county or among those who run its health care institutions. During the 1980s, the five-member county board of supervisors, whose conservative majority has had an enormous impact on health care for the poor, was all male and all white. Successful litigation in 1990 by Mexican-American advocacy groups led to the redrawing of supervisory districts and the election in

1991 of a Latina, the first woman and Latino member to serve on the county board of supervisors. The Los Angeles City Council, which has no direct role in health care programs or institutions, has been more reflective of the city's ethnic and racial composition.

There is no evidence that nonprovider groups have a concerted impact on health care policy in Los Angeles, although the various business and employer organizations are trying to affect public policy at the state level. The labor movement as a whole is only beginning to take a direct interest in health care policy in the state, although public sector employee and health care unions were well represented in Sacramento on these issues throughout most of the 1980s. The poor are represented by a number of advocacy groups, most notably legal aid agencies and coalitions of homeless advocacy and service organizations. Despite some significant victories on behalf of the state's and county's low-income population, these advocates have been more visible than effective in ensuring access to care for the underserved in the face of the persistent underfunding of programs.

Academic medical centers have a large impact on tertiary care; however, they do not dominate hospital or medical care to the same extent as in New York and some other eastern cities. Hospital chains, both investor-owned and not-for-profit, some independent hospitals, medical schools, physicians, insurers, and other provider groups basically operate in a medical care market that is as unfettered by regulation as any in the United States. The constraints placed on these groups and institutions are mainly the result of uncontrolled market forces rather than being political or governmental in nature (even the modest certificate-of-need requirements in California were rescinded in the early 1980s by Governor George Deukmejian). Private providers are buffeted by (1) the large proportion of the population who are uninsured and who generate uncompensated care in hospitals (as well as by hospital behaviors to avoid it), (2) the discount rates negotiated by employers and government payers, (3) the other players in the market, like the supply of nurses and other health workers, and (4) the debt burdens accumulated in the old glory days when hospitals and doctors could more easily dictate terms of reimbursement. All of these forces in the 1990s are converging on what many consider to be a collapsing system of health care.

Costs of Health Care in Los Angeles

In a market economy, competition is supposed to lead to lower costs. In Los Angeles, as in most of the country, despite fierce competition among hospitals, between hospitals and physicians, and among HMOs, PPOs, and other insurers, lower costs did not ensue. Indeed, a major contributing factor to the deterioration of health care in Los Angeles was the substantial increase in costs during the 1980s. Cost increases were especially steep beginning in 1986.

How Costly Is Care in Los Angeles?

For more than two decades, California has spent more money per capita on personal health care than all but two other states. According to data available from the Health Care Financing Administration, the average Californian spends one-fifth more per person on health care than the average American, despite the fact that California has a slightly lower percentage of people over the age of sixty-five. In 1982, the distribution of expenditures in California was somewhat different than for the United States as a whole: California spent a smaller proportion of personal health expenditures on hospitals and nursing homes and more on physician services and dental care. It is reasonable to estimate that California's health expenditures have remained about 20 percent higher than the U.S. average. And it is reasonable to assume that health care costs in Los Angeles are no lower than the California average.

Increases

California's personal health care expenditures increased at about the same rate as national health expenditures from 1966 to 1982. According to one insurance executive, the California "health insurance trend" (which takes into account technology, inflation, the aging of the population, and other factors) showed cost increases of 12–14 percent in 1986, 17 percent in 1987, and 23 percent starting in the middle of 1988. Another insurance CEO provided a similar estimate of costs, noting that the "medical cost trend" in 1988 went up 24 percent.

In general, HMOs that owned their own hospitals and paid physicians on a capitated rate (or salary), like the Kaiser Foundation Health Plan, were able to keep costs under control. However, Los Angeles HMOs that do not own their own hospitals, were, like insurers, faced with substantial price increases. One HMO executive said that in 1987 and 1988, hospital payments went up 10 to 15 percent. In 1988, another HMO faced increases of 10 to 12 percent in inpatient costs and expected 1989 to be worse, with inpatient costs increasing by an additional 10–12 percent and outpatient costs by 15 percent.

Causes

A number of explanations have been given for the increasing expenditures for medical care in the Los Angeles market: the shift from inpatient to outpatient hospital care and the unbundling of hospital outpatient services; the increased utilization of medical care, often referred to as the "insatiable demand" of medical consumers; the growth of medical technology; the aging of the population; the growth of new specialty services, including drug and alcohol treatment and eating-disorder programs; and physician/hospital "greed." Probably, all of these explanations hold some kernel of truth.

From the perspective of insurers and HMOs, the move from inpatient to outpatient services and the "unbundling" of outpatient services were primary reasons for the increasing health care costs. A number of studies have found that the competitive environment fostered by the 1982 reforms in California's health insurance industry (which permitted contracting by health plans for hospital and physician services) and in Medi-Cal (which introduced selective contracting for inpatient care) led to lower inpatient hospital costs than would otherwise have occurred. A study by Melnick and Zwanziger found that the reforms resulted in price competition and declines in the growth rate of inpatient costs and revenues. Further, the degree of competition was directly related to the rate of decline. Another study, by Robinson and Luft, found lower rates of increase in cost per admission for hospitals in competitive markets.

If hospital inpatient costs were finally controlled during the 1980s, the same cannot be said of outpatient costs. As already discussed, hospitals moved many diagnostic and treatment procedures from inpatient to outpatient departments. This shift occurred over a very short period of time. California data show that between 1984 and 1986, the number of knee repair procedures done on an inpatient basis declined 36 percent; hernia repair declined by 59 percent; dilation and curettage (D&C), by 60 percent; tonsillectomy and adenoidectomy, by 31 percent; and lens extraction, by 91 percent. As reported by an insurance executive who had recently worked at Blue Cross of California, the ratio of inpatient/outpatient claims submitted to Blue Cross shifted from 60/40 just a few years ago to 33/67 in 1990.

Costs of outpatient care grew along with the growth in volume. However, according to a number of insurers, volume alone did not explain the steeply rising outpatient costs. As procedures and tests were transferred to the outpatient departments, they were also "unbundled." What had been a single charge on the inpatient side became many charges; the number of "units of service" multiplied. A vice president of HealthMark, an outpatient utilization review firm based in Los Angeles County, commented that hospitals have always billed for outpatient operating room time and anesthesia, but they have recently introduced additional charges for gloves, caps, gowns, masks, and sutures. "They never did surgery before without caps, gloves and gowns," she noted.

As early as the summer of 1986, Los Angeles employers were complaining about rising outpatient costs. One 1985 study of health care costs among nine of southern California's largest employers found that charges for insured services increased by 13 percent overall and that outpatient surgical charges increased by 27 percent. According to one HMO executive, fixed, all-inclusive hospital rates have been going up about 5–10 percent a year, but unbundled outpatient services are increasing by 15–30 percent per year.

Referring to the unbundling and increasing outpatient costs, one insurance executive complained that the "games never end. Charges change constantly and bills are à la carte-d. " The CEO of another HMO, who expected his company's outpatient costs to rise by 15 percent in 1989, explained that outpatient care had become "piece-paid instead of prepaid." He and other HMO and insurance executives stated that they were currently charged more for outpatient surgeries, like D&Cs and cataract removals, than they would have been if the procedures had been done on an inpatient basis. In early 1990, one large suburban Los Angeles hospital billed Medicare $5,300 for a four-hour cataract removal done on an outpatient basis. The physician billed another $3,000.

One CEO was especially angry over his HMO's inability to control emergency room costs: ER patients, he said, are "worked up, worked down, and worked around. Everyone who goes to an emergency room has their financial life in their hands." A 1990 ER bill from a large Los Angeles hospital confirms this observation: The bill for emergency room care for a bad cat scratch requiring six stitches was $487, and the emergency room physician charged over $800, a total of more than $1, 200 for a forty-five-minute visit. Whatever the causes, rising costs are driving changes in the costs and organization of health insurance and in the proportion of the population covered by health insurance.

The Diversification and Decline of Health Insurance

Impact of Health Care Costs
on Insurance Premiums and Access

Higher medical care costs mean higher premiums. As costs of care escalated and a number of insurers and HMOs found that they had set premiums too low and were paying out more than they were taking in, health-benefit premiums were raised accordingly. "When your costs are going up higher than your premiums, you've got to raise the premiums," explained Leonard Schaeffer, president of Blue Cross of California, when he announced large premium increases. Given the large number of insurers, HMOs, and PPOs operating in Los Angeles and the variety of plans offered, information on average premium costs is not available. However, anecdotal evidence and published reports as well as persons interviewed for this study indicate that premiums increased substantially in the latter part of the 1980s. Statewide, health-benefit premium increases in 1988-1989 were often over 20 percent. Two Los Angeles insurance agents reported that health care premiums went up an average of 30 percent in 1988 and another 20 percent in 1989.

Rising costs have made it difficult for small businesses to purchase insurance. The health insurance market in Los Angeles is a "complete disaster," in the opinion of one insurance agent. Although small group insurance is still available, it is too expensive for many small firms. As of January 1990, individual coverage under a Blue Cross health insurance package for a firm of three employees, all in their twenties and healthy, cost, with a $250 deductible and a 20 percent coinsurance rate, between $95 and $100 per month per employee. For family coverage, excluding maternity care, premium costs were $250 per month per employee. With a maternity benefit added, premium costs were $494/month for a childless husband and wife and $574 for a three-person family. These costs were for a young, healthy group. Premium rates were substantially higher for groups with older workers or workers with preexisting health conditions. Finding health insurance for small groups in which one or more members have preexisting conditions is a "major problem," stated one insurance broker.

To make matters worse, the market for small groups is drying up. For example, as of 1990, the Kaiser Foundation Health Plan, the largest HMO in southern California, was limiting enrollment to firms with fifty or more workers. Since 1988, at least thirty-four insurers have stopped selling group policies to small businesses in California.

Premiums for individual health-insurance policies have increased even more than those for group policies. Blue Cross, the state's primary insurer of individuals, has significantly increased the cost of individual policies: "We will no longer be the insurers of last resort in this state," declared Leonard Schaeffer. In 1988, Blue Cross raised the premiums for individual policies by 25 percent: For a single person, an individual policy with a $500 deductible increased to $1,560-$4,440 a year, depending on the subscriber's age; families covered with similar individual deductibles were charged $4,356-$10,188 a year, depending on the age of the head of household. "The whole health insurance system is in serious disarray," said Brent Barnhart of the Association of California Life Insurance Companies. "Even if you take a very healthy person without serious indications of illness, it's not that easy to get good coverage at an affordable price."

Lack of Health Insurance

One out of every three persons in the nonelderly population of Los Angeles is completely uninsured. In 1989, 32 percent of all persons under sixty-five years of age in Los Angeles County were without private or public health insurance coverage—no private health insurance, no Medicare, and no Medicaid coverage—an increase of more than 50 percent since 1979. The lack of insurance among Los Angeles residents is worse than the California average of 23 percent and worse than the U.S. average of 17 percent. The problem is the most severe of all major metropolitan areas in the nation. Among the thirty largest metropolitan areas in the United States, Los Angeles has the largest percentage of nonelderly population who are uninsured. The numbers of uninsured in Los Angeles County are staggering: Some 882,000 children and more than 1.8 million adults in Los Angeles County have no coverage. The uninsured of all ages, nearly 2.7 million people, are without any protection against medical expenses.

Latinos are more than twice as likely to be uninsured as non-Latino whites. In Los Angeles, 48 percent of all Latino children and 51 percent of all Latino nonelderly adults were uninsured in 1989, compared to 19 percent of non-Latino white children and adults.

Low-income people are far more likely to be uninsured than are more affluent people. In Los Angeles, nearly half of all poor children (44 percent) and half of those who are near poor (51 percent) are without insurance or Medicaid coverage. Among nonelderly adults in Los Angeles, 57 percent of the poor and near poor are uninsured. But lack of health insurance coverage is not a problem of poor people alone. Among those with family incomes at least 300 percent of the poverty level, 18 percent of children and 16 percent of nonelderly adults are without any coverage.

According to state data, in FY 1978-79, 14 percent of the county's population was enrolled in Medi-Cal. By 1987, as a result of eligibility cutbacks in the Medi-Cal program, the county's Medi-Cal population had declined to 10 percent. It is likely that this percentage has increased with the passage of federal legislation providing Medicaid for all poor pregnant women and emergency patients regardless of immigration status and with the passage of the Immigration Reform and Control Act of 1987, which provides Medicaid coverage for immigrant children and the elderly who have been granted amnesty.

One of the main factors contributing to the magnitude of the uninsured population is the large proportion of employees who do not receive health insurance as a fringe benefit from their employers. Although 70 percent of full-time full-year employees in California receive health insurance as a fringe benefit, 16 percent are left completely uninsured; they are not covered by health insurance as a fringe benefit, nor are they covered by another family member's job-related insurance or by any other coverage. Only half of all full-time part-year employees (50 percent) and part-time employees (53 percent) have employment-based health insurance (through their own or a family member's job), and one in every three full-time part-year employees (31 percent) and one in four part-time employees (24 percent) remain completely uninsured.

Relatively large percentages of employees do not receive health insurance as a fringe benefit in retail businesses and service firms—the high-growth sectors of the labor market—and in some nondurable-goods manufacturing firms. For example, two thirds of the more than 80,000 garment industry workers in Los Angeles are completely uninsured.

Latino employees are more than twice as likely to be uninsured as employees who are non-Latino whites, blacks, and members of other ethnic groups. Latino workers—even those who work full-time full-year—are far less likely to receive health insurance as a subsidized fringe benefit than are members of other ethnic groups mainly because a large proportion work in small firms and in industries that do not provide health insurance.

Lack of health insurance is a serious personal problem for the uninsured and a significant social problem for the entire community and state. The uninsured add substantial costs to the uncompensated-care burden of hospitals, creating financial pressures on county hospitals, many not-for-profit hospitals, and community clinics. In FY 1984-85, California's hospitals reported uncompensated care (bad debts and charity care) totaling $1.1 billion, with county hospitals accounting for half the total and four times their share of all hospital beds. The provision of just the most essential health care needs of low-income uninsured people thus adds to the fiscal difficulties of the counties and the state. This problem is likely to worsen as the number of AIDS patients, including those who are medically indigent, increases during the next few years. The large number of uninsured persons who end up in emergency rooms has forced several Los Angeles hospitals to withdraw from the county's trauma care network.

In sum, Los Angeles is a relatively affluent metropolitan area, but that affluence is unevenly distributed. Large numbers of people are poor or near poor, and many are without any protection against health care expenses. Their access to care is thus greatly reduced. When they do obtain medical care, the costs of their care add to Los Angeles County's fiscal crisis and to the burden on taxpayers. The cost of services they receive from private hospitals is added to the premiums of privately insured patients and strains the financial viability of those hospitals that try to meet community needs for maternity, emergency, and trauma care.

Insurers, HMOs, and PPOs

Despite the large number of uninsured people in Los Angeles, two-thirds of the population still have some form of coverage, and 60 percent are covered by private insurance. Within the private insurance industry, alternative delivery systems (ADSs)—HMOs, PPOs, and their hybrids— were virtually born in California. Beginning with the establishment of the Ross-Loos Health Plan in 1929 and the Kaiser Foundation Health Plan in 1945, and continuing with the 1982 California reform legislation authorizing preferred provider organizations (PPOs), the California environment has proved receptive to innovations in the delivery of health care. The administratively complex, costly, and almost chaotic health care system in Los Angeles cannot be understood without examining the growth of ADSs during the 1980s and their impact on traditional health insurers.

The "Growth of Weird and New Things." Following the enactment of the 1982 reform legislation, PPOs sprang into existence virtually overnight. Almost every group imaginable got into the act: California PPOs are sponsored by hospitals, physicians, other health providers, physician independent practice associations, foundations, entrepreneurs, independent administrator service organizations, insurance companies, and employer and union trusts.

PPOs are unregulated, and their growth cannot be measured accurately. However, both published and anecdotal sources reveal that PPOs have undergone vertiginous expansion since the early 1980s. The number of PPOs responding to an annual California survey conducted for the California Association of Hospitals and Health Systems (CAHHS) grew from thirty-seven in 1984 to seventy-two in 1988. One insurance executive interviewed for this report estimates that there are 120 PPOs operating in the state.

According to estimates by the seventy-two PPOs responding to the CAHHS survey, over 16 million Californians have the option of enrolling in a PPO and over 9 million have done so. California PPOs have signed 4,957 hospital contracts and 339,063 physician contracts.

During the 1980s, the number of HMOs and their members also grew prodigiously. In 1988, California had fifty-three HMOs operating within its borders; fifteen of these operated out of the Los Angeles area, and an additional nine marketed in Los Angeles. Of these twenty-four HMOs, ten began operations in the 1980s. More than 4 million persons were enrolled in seventeen Los Angeles–based HMOs by July 1989.

In addition to the HMOs and PPOs operating in Los Angeles, a hybrid of these organizational forms began doing business in the latter part of the 1980s. A number of insurers offer enrollees the choice of seeking care through their HMOs or PPOs and switching back and forth at will. Indeed, the variety of plans offering different and often overlapping organizational arrangements can be confusing. For example, under its "Group Products," Blue Cross of California offers a Fee-For-Service (FFS) Indemnity Plan; Prudent Buyer (PPO); CaliforniaCare (nonfederally qualified

HMO), TakeCare (federally qualified HMO), and Option Plus, a triple-option plan that offers subscribers the choice of an HMO (CaliforniaCare), a PPO (Prudent Buyer), and an FFS. Under its "Individual Products," Blue Cross offers Personal Prudent Buyer (PPO), Basic Major Protection (FFS), CompanionCare Plan (FFS), CommuniCare (Capitated), UltraCare (FFS), and SeniorCare (FFS).

Finally, traditional indemnity plans continue to offer fee-for-service insurance. Data on the market penetration of indemnity plans are not available. One insurance company CEO estimated that in 1984, the market was 75 percent indemnity and 25 percent HMO/PPO. In 1989, he said, it was the reverse. He commented that during five short years we have seen the "growth of weird and new things" that have "splintered the market."

"Cutthroat" Competition. During the 1980s, competition within the insurance/HMO industry was, if anything, more intense than in the hospital industry. "Competition is as cutthroat in Los Angeles County as anywhere in the country. It is fierce, relentless, suicidal," complained one CEO. This competition led to a price war among HMOs and PPOs. At least two HMO executives interviewed for this study accused private insurers of pricing their PPO products "lower than cost" in order to drive HMOs out of the market: "Insurers, because of their larger asset base, tried to starve the competition," said one HMO executive. Echoing this sentiment, another HMO executive explained that PPOs were the indemnity insurers' way to "capture the market from HMOs." Robert Gumbiner, chairman and CEO of FHP Inc., a large, successful Los Angeles–based HMO, compared the actions of the insurers to John D. Rockefeller's successful efforts to corner the oil market: "Maybe the insurance companies are just trying to buy businesses until they drive small- and medium-size HMOs out. . . . I don't know what their strategy is. . . . How can their strategy be to lose millions of dollars every year forever?"

Los Angeles insurance executives disagreed with this assessment. "Everyone priced wrong," responded one CEO. Another explained that one insurer who faced substantial losses during the late 1980s had simply "mispriced" its product and made a "mistake." Some insurers also accused HMOs of undercutting the competition by setting artificially low prices. In one article, California Blue Cross's financial difficulties were explained this way: "Increasingly, Blue Cross is finding itself squeezed between other giants like Maxicare and Kaiser-Permanente, who are trying to improve their market share, and aggressive newcomers with hot plans at 'loss-leader' prices."

Whether insurers priced below cost by design or "mistake, " the price competition in 1986-1987 and poor business decisions by a number of insurers and HMOs left the insurance industry fiscally shaken. Blue Cross of California lost $55.4 million in 1986 and nearly $100 million in the first half of 1987. As one HMO executive put it, Blue Cross was more "red than blue."

A number of HMOs also found themselves in difficult financial straits in the late 1980s. Health Net, a large HMO that broke off from Blue Cross in 1985, "lost money hand over fist," reported one insurance executive. Two other major Los Angeles–based HMOs—Maxicare, serving a large privately insured population, and United Health Plan, an HMO that marketed primarily to the low-income and minority communities of Los Angeles through Medi-Cal and Medicare enrollment—declared bankruptcy in that year. The financial problems of both HMOs seemed to be more the result of poor management than of the competitive environment of Los Angeles. United Health Plan survived seventeen months of Chapter 11 reorganization.

If some HMOs fared poorly, others thrived. Kaiser-Permanente Medical Care Program of Southern California, which provides care to all of the state's southern counties (including Los Angeles, Orange, and San Diego), added over 400 beds and grew from 1.56 million to 1.9 million members from 1980 through 1988. FHP also fared well. In the fiscal year ending June 1988, the company earned $16.5 million on revenue of $503.5 million. Much of FHP's growth came from Medicare enrollment, which increased 43 percent in FY 1988 alone; in 1988 Medicare enrollees made up over 27 percent of the plan's membership. PacificCare, another large, southern California HMO, has also done well by its Medicare contract. Medicare accounts for about 25 percent of the plan's membership, and it provides more than half of its revenues.

And the Poor. Although some HMOs were able to do well on Medicare enrollees, they did not accommodate the Medi-Cal population well. Few HMOs in Los Angeles accept Medi-Cal capitated enrollees, and most of those that do strictly limit enrollment. Kaiser-Permanente of Southern California, for example, enrolls only 24,000 Medi-Cal recipients out of a total membership of 1.9 million. In all, only nine of the twenty-four HMOs that market in Los Angeles accept Medi-Cal enrollees.

The growth of HMOs and PPOs and the competitive Los Angeles market left the poor with few health care options. Today, neither HMOs nor PPOs subsidize care for the uninsured poor. Moreover, the poor on Medi-Cal have little access to HMOs and access to PPOs.

The Public Sector

Who Cares for the Poor?

The uninsured poor and near poor—915, 000 in Los Angeles—get care where they can find it. Many receive care from private hospitals, which provided $507 million of uncompensated care in California in 1985-1986.

Many also are treated at the forty free and community clinics in Los Angeles County. Services provided by these clinics are critical to the thousands of poor who get through their doors. However, these facilities are overwhelmed with patients and are limited in the kinds of specialty care they can provide. For example, the Venice Family Clinic, which serves a largely undocumented Latino population and the homeless on the west side of Los Angeles, received 31,000 patient visits in 1989, a 21 percent increase over the previous year. Yet, the clinic still must turn away 5,000 people a year for lack of space.

The predominant share of subsidized care for the uninsured poor as well as for a large proportion of Medi-Cal patients is provided by the Los Angeles County Department of Health Services. Los Angeles County began providing care to its indigent population in 1878 with the construction of its first hospital. Today the county operates the second largest local public health system in the nation, with six hospitals, more than 4,300 licensed beds, forty-one health centers and subcenters, and five comprehensive health centers. These hospitals and clinics provide nearly 1 million inpatient days, approximately 3 million outpatient visits, and 400,000 emergency room visits per year to the poor of Los Angeles. The Department of Health Services (DHS) is the largest county department; in FY 1987-88, it had 23,097 budgeted positions and an operating budget of $1.3 billion.

Public Hospitals and Clinics

In California, as throughout the United States, health care for the uninsured poor is the responsibility of local government. California state law requires the counties to "relieve and support" their indigent residents. Although Los Angeles County's four acute-care hospitals, one rehabilitation hospital, one nursing home facility, and its clinics and comprehensive health centers are geographically dispersed throughout the county, they are inadequate to meet the needs of the tens of thousands of poor people seeking care. Too few resources and too little money collide with overwhelming need at county hospitals and health centers, with the result being long delays in obtaining care and an undermining of the ability of staff to provide quality services.

The growth of the uninsured population in the 1980s strained county resources. From FY 1981-82 through FY 1988-89, the number of public hospital admissions increased by 32 percent; average daily admissions, 20 percent; ambulatory care visits, 63 percent; public health visits, 32 percent; emergency room visits, 31 percent; DHS hospital births, 63 percent; contract hospital births (county-paid deliveries in private hospitals), 252 percent; and total hospital births, 80 percent.

Financing

During the 1980s, the lack of adequate financing for indigent health care in Los Angeles County led to one fiscal crisis after another. Neither state nor county funds were adequate to meet the growing demand for county services.

Declining State and County Spending. Proposition 13, passed by the voters in 1978, and the health care reform legislation of 1982 changed the health care delivery system in California, unleashing fierce competition among hospitals for privately insured patients and, over the decade of the 1980s, undermining care to the state's poor and uninsured populations. Proposition 13 reduced the tax revenues of the local governments by 40 percent, which sharply curtailed their ability to provide public services, including health care. The initiative also restricted the future growth of tax revenues by requiring a two-thirds vote of the legislature for new state taxes and a two-thirds vote of the local electorate to raise local special taxes. Although state "bail-out" bills created a County Health Services Fund to replace property tax money previously used by counties to meet public health and indigent care responsibilities, state money was not enough to meet indigent care needs as they increased during the 1980s.

Proposition 13 was a major tremor felt by local county governments responsible for indigent care but was largely ignored by the private health care sector. The reform legislation of 1982 was different, setting off shock waves that transformed both the private and public health care landscapes. The 1982 reforms were as extraordinary as the process that gave birth to them. Faced with a massive budget deficit, a select group of Democratic and Republican legislators went behind closed doors (where the lobbyists could not get to them) and emerged after a weekend of negotiations with a legislative package that cut the Medi-Cal budget by 10 percent (approximately $.5 billion) and allowed both the Medi-Cal program and private insurers to contract with hospitals for predetermined reimbursement rates.

Specifically, the 1982 legislation dropped 270,000 medically indigent adults (MIAs) from the Medi-Cal program. Counties were given responsibility to provide services to the MIAs, but they were provided with only 70 percent of the dollars the state would have spent on this population under Medi-Cal. Equally important, the legislation allowed Medi-Cal to "selectively contract" with hospitals to serve the Medi-Cal population and permitted private insurers to form preferred provider organizations (PPOs) to negotiate reduced-cost hospital and physician contracts.

In the ensuing decade, the Medi-Cal cutbacks and reforms, especially the dumping of the MIAs from Medi-Cal, led to a diminution of care to the state's indigent population, and the private insurance reforms produced what many hospitals and insurers have found to be a competitive and administrative nightmare. Medi-Cal imposed selective contracting and discount rates on hospitals just before Medicare introduced PPS, a double whammy from the perspective of hospitals that had grown comfortable with virtually unlimited reimbursement for their expenditures. Nowhere has the impact of the 1982 health care legislation been more dramatic than in Los Angeles County.

Proposition 13 sharply reduced the tax revenues of the local governments. In response, the state legislature authorized the County Health Services Fund to provide matching funds to counties for their indigent health care programs. In 1983, these funds were supplemented by funds from the Medically Indigent Services Program (MISP) in order to compensate the counties for care provided to the medically indigent adults who were dropped from the Medi-Cal program and added to the counties' responsibilities.

When the state shifted responsibility for 270,000 MIAs, including 80,000 in Los Angeles, to the counties in 1982, it agreed to provide the counties with 70 percent of the dollars it would have spent had the MIAs remained in the Medi-Cal program. This support has fallen to about 55 percent as a result of Governor Deukmejian's vetoes of increased appropriations for the MIA program and for county health services generally. Neither the County Health Services Fund nor MISP has provided adequate cost-of-living adjustments (COLAs). For FY 1988-89, for example, inadequate COLAs for the County Health Services Fund and MISP resulted in a drop in their real (inflation adjusted) contributions to the Los Angeles County system of $55.7 million and $93.6 million, respectively.

Like the state, Los Angeles County also has not maintained its commitment to indigent health care. The five-member board of supervisors, which was controlled by a conservative three-member majority from 1981 to 1991, voted year after year to reduce county health care services. The county's contribution to the Department of Health Services' budget declined from 16.8 percent of the county's total available funding in FY 1980-81 to 10.6 percent for FY 1988-89 and to only 8 percent in FY 1989-90. The county's $246.9 million contribution to the Department of Health Services in FY 1988-89 was only $4.9 million more than in FY 1980-81.

This pattern prevailed in California throughout the 1980s. State and county spending for the medically indigent population did not keep up with the growth of the uninsured low-income population and with inflation. Between 1983 and 1986, the number of uninsured poor and near-poor people in California grew 10.9 percent, but after adjusting for inflation, total state and county spending for indigent medical care increased less than 1 percent. As a consequence, inflation-adjusted public spending per medically indigent person in California fell 9 percent in just those three years.

County Charges and the Ability-to-Pay Plans. In part to make up for declining revenues and in part because of a political belief that everyone should pay something for health care, the Los Angeles Board of Supervisors instituted a new policy in 1981 of charging uninsured patients $20 per county clinic visit and $25 per county hospital outpatient visit. Uninsured inpatients at county hospitals were also asked to pay a portion of their bill. County charges for outpatient visits, including those for the first seven prenatal care visits, have since increased to $35 at public health centers and comprehensive health centers, $40 at county hospital outpatient clinics, $45 at comprehensive health center urgent-care centers, and $60 at county hospital emergency rooms. For women delivering their babies at county hospitals, the fee is $800.

At the same time that the charges were introduced, the county instituted an ability-to-pay (ATP) plan for uninsured indigent patients who were unable to pay the county's charges. In 1989, a family of four could have an income of no more than $1,401/month to be eligible for ATP clinic services and $1,116/month for ATP hospital care.

Although the ATP policy looks good on paper, it has been inadequately implemented and large numbers of poor people in Los Angeles County have not gotten the free or reduced cost care for which they are eligible. One study of ATP implementation found that patients were not being informed about the program.

Despite successful litigation against the county by Los Angeles Legal Services programs because of the faulty implementation of the ATP program, the county Department of Health Services continues to place substantial barriers in the way of poor county patients in need of ATP. A court-mandated monitoring study of the ATP program found that in 1989, 38 percent of county patients said they never received an ATP notice; only 17 percent of all people calling county clinics and 6 percent of all Spanish-speaking people calling the clinics were given a minimum amount of information on the program; 72 percent of callers to county clinics were informed about the county charge policy but not about ATP; and scheduling an appointment for ATP was very difficult.

The county's charge policy primarily affects poor Latino immigrants, who are often afraid to apply for public assistance, including ATP and Medi-Cal, or who cannot manage to get through the county bureaucracy. The fears of the Latino population, especially the undocumented community, have been justified. Twice during the 1980s, in 1981 and again in 1986, the county board of supervisors voted to require all persons seeking county health services to either apply for Medi-Cal or pay the county fee out-of-pocket. These policies literally forced undocumented immigrants to pay for services because, until recently, Medi-Cal applications were screened by the Immigration and Naturalization Service. One unpublished county report stated that 82 percent of women (the majority of whom were Latinas) receiving prenatal care at county facilities paid up-front for that care.

Surveys of county patients and studies of the impact of the charge poli-cies for prenatal care and sexually transmitted disease (STD) visits show that the fees keep large numbers of indigent county residents from obtain-ing needed health care. One public health nurse, who recently worked for the county, remembers seeing pregnant women who did not have Medi-Cal being "harassed and embarrassed" to pay. When she would visit pregnant women to find out why they did not come for their follow-up appointments, they responded that "they didn't have any money." "The women learned that they had to have the money."

Closures, Cutbacks, and Understaffing

In 1981, the same year the new board of supervisors adopted the coun-ty's charge policies, the board, in a "significant departure for DHS and the county," closed eight health subcenters. Since then, the number of addi-tional facility closures, while devastating, has not been that great. In the early 1980s, the county closed its Long Beach hospital, which had been used primarily for long-term care. In 1989, the county, responding to ve-toes of funds by Governor Deukmejian, also closed three mental health clinics as well as thirteen family planning clinics. During the 1980s, how-ever, the county also opened up a rebuilt Olive View Hospital that had been destroyed in the 1971 earthquake.

Annual, seemingly inexorable cutbacks in county services during the 1980s, rather than facility closures, have severely limited the ability of the Department of Health Services to provide health services to the county's poor. From 1980 to 1990, the county's health care system was literally starved for capital and equipment as well as for personnel.

The county's health care physical plant and equipment have been al-lowed to deteriorate. The Department of Health Services' rate of invest-ment is 0.7 percent, compared to a rate of 8.8 percent for all California hos-pitals. The contrast between what the county spends for capital and equipment for its hospitals and what private hospitals in the community spend is dramatic. In the last four quarters ending September 30, 1988, Los Angeles County spent the following on its acute care hospitals: $1.66 mil-lion on 501-bed Harbor/UCLA Medical Center; $159,000 on 410-bed Mar-tin Luther King (MLK) Hospital; $1.78 million on 1,436-bed L.A. County/USC (LAC/USC) Medical Center; and $4.59 million on the newly opened 235-bed Olive View Hospital. By comparison, Cedars-Sinai Hospital (1,005 beds) spent $21.6 million; Centinela Hospital (378 beds), $11.46 mil-lion; UCLA Medical Center (586 beds), $35.5 million; and Northridge Medical Center (345 beds), $9.95 million. These private and university hospital expenditures were typical of what was spent by noncounty hospitals.

The DHS is well aware of the state of its physical plant. In a 1989 letter to the board of supervisors protesting planned reductions in county spending, Robert Gates, director of DHS, wrote that "many of our facilities have deteriorated to the point of needing replacement. We have identified needed capital projects totalling more than $1 billion." According to Jerry Buckingham, director of LAC/USC Medical Center, "The infrastructure is coming apart."

Equipment has also been allowed to fall into disrepair. Reports by Los Angeles Legal Services programs on quality of care in the public hospital system in 1987 and again in 1989 quote scores of complaints by doctors and nurses about lack of equipment and outdated equipment. The county hospitals do not have enough CAT scanners, heart monitors, Harvard pumps, mammography units, gurneys, wheelchairs, and other basic equipment required in modern American hospitals. Lack of equipment, said a former nurse at the LAC/USC AIDS program, means that it can take six to eight weeks for patients to receive essential diagnostic tests such as CAT scans.

Perhaps the gravest problem in the county's health care system is not crumbling physical plants or equipment shortages but lack of staff. Nursing shortages threaten the county's ability to provide decent health care. In 1989, the DHS had approximately 800 budgeted, vacant RN positions. There are also shortages in electrocardiograph (EKG) technicians, physical therapists, clerical support staff, interpreters, and sanitarians.

Quality of Care

Quality of care in the health care system of Los Angeles County has been severely compromised by too many patients, lack of equipment and staff, and inadequate physical plants. By any measure of quality—structure, process, outcome—the county's public hospitals fare poorly.

The entire county health care system is overwhelmed with patients. The number of facilities—inpatient, outpatient, and clinic—is grossly inadequate to meet the needs of so many uninsured county residents. Although hospitals in the county operate, overall, at 61 percent occupancy, the county's four acute-care hospitals average 85 percent occupancy for staffed beds. In reality, DHS hospitals often operate at over 100 percent occupancy of staffed beds. It is not uncommon for women to be delivered in hallways; for the fire marshal to close L.A. County/USC Hospital to new admissions because beds in the hallways pose a fire hazard; for emergency patients to "wait days on gurneys" or for ERs to be "overflowing with patients needing critical care beds, who often wait as long as three days in the emergency room"; for cardiac patients to "wait two to five days for a monitored bed to open up"; for ICU patients to be prematurely bumped back to the wards; and for women who have just given birth to "sit in wheelchairs for several hours" or "be sent home six to eight hours after delivery without their babies" because of a lack of postpartum beds. Physicians and nurses at DHS facilities say that the average wait for a mammogram appointment at an outpatient clinic is three months; for an initial specialty care appointment, two months; for a chest x-ray, two months; for a diabetes appointment, two or three months; for an initial appointment in a neurology clinic, three months; and for a gynecology appointment, three months. The beds that are available for patients are inadequately staffed. In 1988, after describing in long detail the problems of staffing for the obstetrical ward at LAC/USC, one county nurse wrote, "how can this hospital be adhering to JCAHO standards for patient care [with] everyday conditions like this?"

In fact, the county does not adhere to the standards of either the Joint Commission on Accreditation of Healthcare Organizations (JCAHO) or the state Department of Health Services' Licensing and Certification Division. For example, during one survey of LAC/USC by the Licensing and Certification Division, the surveyors found that the "nursing staff is very visibly insufficient." A joint state-JCAHO survey of Martin Luther King Hospital (MLK) in June 1989 found such serious deficiencies that the hospital was threatened with loss of its JCAHO accreditation. The survey team found a "consistent shortage of registered nurses. Care assignment was given in many instances to personnel not qualified nor trained to provide professional nursing care." In addition, one surgical unit that required six RNs had only one RN on one of the seven days reviewed and had two RNs on the other six days. These nurses were expected to care for thirty or more surgical patients.

The state also cited MLK because of a major breakdown in several areas of patient care, including quality assurance, infection control, nursing, and dietary services. Moreover, surveyors found that equipment had fallen into disrepair, drugs were left unattended, patient records were misfiled, and inexperienced nursing students cared for acutely ill patients. The county and the hospital were able to stave off the denial of Medicare and Medicaid reimbursement when the hospital passed a follow-up inspection less than three months later. To pass this inspection, the hospital closed four wards and hired 200 additional employees.

The lack of staff, equipment, and supervision compromises the process of care for the county's indigents. In a searing exposé published just prior to the MLK inspection, the *Los Angeles Times* described several examples of grossly unacceptable quality of care at the hospital, the lack of any quality assessment system, and inadequate supervision by full-time staff, who charged the hospital for time spent in their private practices. The *Times* also found that the rate of emergency room deaths at MLK and the hospital's nosocomial infection rate were significantly greater than at the DHS's other acute-care hospitals.

MLK's quality-of-care problems are reflected in its mortality data. Although mortality data should not be used as the only measure of quality, they may, combined with other criteria, indicate quality-of-care deficiencies. Between 1986 and 1988, MLK had the worst Medicare mortality rate in California and one of the fifty worst rates nationally: 22.7 percent of all Medicare patients died within thirty days of hospital admission, a rate 54.4 percent higher than expected. MLK also had the state's highest standardized death rate for newborn babies in 1986, according to a sophisticated analysis of perinatal death-rate data by researchers at the University of California at Santa Barbara. The hospital's newborn death rate of 17 per 1,000 live births was 37 percent higher than expected when compared to the statewide average. The analysis takes into account the infant's birth weight, sex, and race as well as multiple births. L.A. County/USC Medical Center had a standardized newborn death rate that was 21 percent greater than expected.

Access to care for the poor of Los Angeles suffered devastating setbacks during the 1980s due to lack of DHS oversight; to a board of supervisors that paid scant attention to the problems of the county's hospitals and clinics, except to complain about state funding and propose service cutbacks; to a generally indifferent populace; and to a private health care system that made systematic efforts to reduce its uncompensated-care load. The county and especially its large low-income population have paid for this neglect in increased infant death rates, a rise in communicable diseases, a lack of initiative to prevent the spread of AIDS and treat AIDS patients, and gross neglect of the county's severely mentally ill, many of whom roam the streets of Los Angeles.

Access

Persons interviewed for this study spoke of a health care system for the poor that was on the verge of collapse. Although few studies have been done to assess systematically the health care problems in Los Angeles, anecdotal reports by DHS staff of the long waits patients experience to get into the county system as well as county documents on waiting times for specialty appointments support the assessment that the delivery of health care for both Medi-Cal and uninsured patients is in critical condition.

Despite their coverage, Medi-Cal patients in Los Angeles and throughout California often are unable to find physicians willing to treat them. For example, in 1985, there were only 265 obstetrics-gynecology (OB-GYN) providers in Los Angeles County who would accept Medi-Cal patients, a ratio of one provider for every 664 Medi-Cal-eligible woman of child-bearing age. Moreover, many of these providers strictly limit their practices. Because they lack access to private providers, an increasing number of Medi-Cal patients, especially obstetrical patients, are going to overcrowded county facilities. In 1987, 74 percent of all Medi-Cal inpatient hospital reimbursement and 54 percent of hospital outpatient reimbursement went to DHS hospitals.

Yet, Medi-Cal patients still have access to the private sector. The same is not true of the uninsured. In Los Angeles, as throughout the state, a vast difference exists between access to care for the uninsured and access for the Medi-Cal population. For example, researchers at the UCLA Medical Center studied a group of medically indigent adults (MIAs) who lost their Medi-Cal eligibility when, in 1982, the MIAs were dropped from Medi-Cal and had to depend on county health services. The researchers also followed a comparison group of Medi-Cal patients who did not lose their Medi-Cal eligibility. Six months and one year after the MIAs lost their Medi-Cal coverage, they were in significantly poorer health and had less access to health services than before they lost Medi-Cal and in comparison to the patients who were still on Medi-Cal. Hypertension among MIAs was significantly worse; their diabetes was less well controlled; and several patients died under circumstances that could be attributed to loss of coverage for needed care and medications. The authors concluded that the elevated blood pressure among the MIAs at six months increased their relative risk of dying by 40 percent.

The Public's Health and Public Health Care Services

Perinatal Care and Infant Mortality. A third of all California babies are born in Los Angeles County. Of all pregnant women in the county, one-fourth seek care from the county Department of Health Services. Often, that care is inadequate. Throughout the 1980s, the DHS was unable to keep up with the growing demand for perinatal services. In 1986, 17.3 percent of women who delivered their babies at DHS facilities received late (last trimester) or no prenatal care. In 1987, 24 percent, and in the first half of 1988, 27 percent to 30 percent, of women delivering at MLK received no prenatal care at all. In affluent areas of Los Angeles, such as the Westside and Malibu, over 80 percent of pregnant women begin prenatal care in the first trimester. In poor neighborhoods of south-central Los Angeles, less than 60 percent of women begin prenatal care during the first three months of pregnancy. Data for 1988 showed that whereas, overall, one in four pregnant women in Los Angeles did not begin prenatal care in the first trimester, for black and Latino women the rates were 32 percent and 38 percent, respectively.

One reason women have given for not seeking prenatal care is the county's charge policies. In one survey, over 57 percent of women who delivered at DHS hospitals without having received prenatal care said that the care was "unaffordable."

Other women do not receive care because they cannot get appointments. As the number of uninsured poor women seeking care at Los Angeles County DHS facilities grew, so did the waits for prenatal care appointments. In 1987, for example, of twenty-five clinics studied, eighteen had waiting periods for an intake appointment of four weeks or longer; ten of six weeks or longer; five, of eight weeks or longer; and at one center, women calling for appointments were told they would have to wait twelve weeks. In 1986, 2.8 percent of white pregnant women in the county received late or no prenatal care, compared to 7.5 percent of black women and 8.3 percent of white Latino women.

DHS hospitals as well as clinics are overwhelmed by the large number of pregnant uninsured women in the county. One out of every 200 infants born in the United States is born at LAC/USC Medical Center's Women's Hospital. In FY 1988-89, 38,000 babies were delivered at DHS hospitals, a system that can "safely" deliver 35,000 babies, according to DHS director, Robert Gates. As many as 45,000 infants were expected to be born in county facilities during FY 1989-90. County obstetricians have angrily protested the "battlefront obstetrics" being practiced at Women's Hospital.

Inadequate access to prenatal care coupled with an alarming rise in crack cocaine use in poor minority communities and few drug treatment programs for drug-addicted mothers have predictably resulted in an increase in low-birth-weight babies and newborn deaths. Between 1987 and 1988, the percent of babies born weighing less than 2,500 grams, or 5.5 pounds, increased by 17 percent (from 5.3 percent in 1987 to 6.2 percent in 1988); in 1988, 13.7 percent of black babies were born with low birth weights, a 32 percent increase from the previous year (see Table 4. 1).

Along with the increased number of babies born with low birth weights, the county's infant mortality rate rose from 8.2 deaths per 1, 000 live births in 1987 to 9.6 deaths in 1988. Although the white infant mortality rate decreased from 10.0 to 8.8 deaths per 1, 000 live births (a 12 percent decline), the Latino rate rose from 8.2 to 9.6 (a 17 percent rise) and the black rate jumped from 16.3 to 21.1—a 29 percent increase (see Table 4.1).

Mental Health. During the 1980s, the county's mental health system for the poor was, like the acute-care system, unable to meet the need for services. A gross shortage of county mental health beds and reductions in the number of county-funded mental health clinics has left the system unable to provide even basic mental health services. County DHS hospitals have only 1, 080 mental health beds, one-fourth the number in New York City public hospitals. A 1988 grand jury investigation found that 50 percent of

TABLE 4.1   Infant Mortality by Ethnic Group in Los Angeles County, 1987 and 1988

Infant Mortality (deaths/1,000 live births)	*1987*	*1988*	*Percent Change*
White Anglo	10.0	8.8	−12%
Black	16.3	21.1	+29%
Latino	5.8	7.5	+29%
All Births	8.2	9.6	+17%
U.S. Average	10.1		

Source: J. Scott, "Rise in Infant Deaths Laid to Drugs, Prenatal Neglect," *Los Angeles Times,* February 3, 1990, pp. A1, A33.

those seeking admission to mental health facilities are routinely turned away because of the bed shortage.

In 1987, a coalition of county physicians and managers issued a report describing conditions at county mental health facilities: "On every side, restriction and entrenchments have made conditions intolerably bad . . . patients in dire need of emergency services are being turned away daily." Referring to the lack of beds for the mentally ill, the chairman of the psychiatry department at Harbor/UCLA Medical Center said, "We play a game of 'Sophie's choice' night after night after night. It's a horrible job." Neither the county nor the state is willing to fund mental health services adequately. In 1989, a shortfall in state health care funding led the county board of supervisors to close five Department of Mental Health clinics and cut services at seven others. Today, only the most severely mentally ill have any access at all to county-funded outpatient care. The executive director of one of the remaining county mental health clinics said, "We are looking at this point at a complete and utter disaster in the mental health system. The mental health system has gone insane."

AIDS. The AIDS epidemic in Los Angeles shows no signs of abating. In 1990 an estimated 112,000 residents of the county were infected with the HIV virus, and between January and November 1989, 2, 274 newly diagnosed AIDS cases were reported in the county, a 28 percent increase from the comparable period a year earlier. As of September 30, 1989, 8,063 cases of AIDS were reported, and 5,306 persons had died of the disease. AIDS in Los Angeles is still predominantly a disease among white homosexual and bisexual males. Through September 1989, 65 percent of AIDS cases were white, 16 percent were black, and 18 percent were Latino. (For reported AIDS cases through June 1989, see Table 4.2.)

However, AIDS is spreading swiftly in the county's large Latino population. In the first half of 1989, 24 percent of the newly diagnosed AIDS cases were Latino, up from 16 percent in 1986. The large number of poorly educated, undocumented immigrants in the Los Angeles area, many of whom are fearful of contact with government agencies and have strong re-

TABLE 4.2　Reported AIDS Cases by Exposure Group, Ethnicity, and Year of Diagnosis, Los Angeles County, 1984–1989

	Percent					
Exposure Category	1984	1985	1986	1987	1988	1989*
Adults						
Homosexual/bisexual male contact	80	85	85	81	78	79
IV drug user (IVDU)	2	3	2	4	6	5
Homosexual/bisexual IVDU	13	6	6	8	8	9
Other	4	7	6	8	8	7
Total	817	900	1,424	1,823	1,738	636
Children						
Hemophilia or coagulation disorder	0	0	0	8	21	0
Parent with or at risk of AIDS	33	25	67	50	43	80
Transfusion recipient	67	75	33	42	36	20
Total children	9	12	9	12	14	10
Total number	826	912	1,433	1,835	1,752	646

*Reported cases through June 1989.
Source: Los Angeles County Department of Health Services, Memoranda of Robert Gates, Director of Health Services, to Los Angeles County Board of Supervisors, "AIDS—Report for June 1989," July 17, 1989.

ligious sanctions against discussing homosexuality and sexual behavior, have helped spread the disease among poor Latinos. The director of the Gay and Lesbian Community Services Center reported seeing a great many more HIV-infected gay Latinos than gay whites coming to his clinic: "In the past two months, our clinic has found 45 percent [infection rates] among gay and bisexual Latinos," compared to 17 percent among Anglo gays. "This figure just leaps out at you.... It is really alarming."

AIDS is also spreading among the heterosexual contacts of HIV-infected drug abusers. Although women made up only 3 percent of persons with AIDS in Los Angeles in the late 1980s, the disease has been infecting groups of young women, called "strawberries," who exchange sex for cocaine, according to Dr. Shirley Fanin, head of the county's Communicable Disease Control Programs.

Denial, apathy, and hostility have all played a role in the county's lackluster performance in fighting the spread of AIDS and caring for its victims: The Catholic archbishop of Los Angeles has taken a strong stand against the use of condoms; when asked for help in "adopting" an AIDS patient, only 10 percent of the county's black ministers responded; only three Latino doctors attended a county-sponsored forum for Latino doctors on treating AIDS and HIV infection; the conservative majority on the board of supervisors has twice voted against programs to distribute bleach to IV drug users; and, with the exception of the entertainment industry, the business community has provided almost no AIDS funding.

Lack of support from the Los Angeles Board of Supervisors has severely hampered efforts to control the AIDS epidemic. Members of the AIDS leadership community in the county unanimously condemn the board for its lack of leadership: "Under the present political philosophy of the board, we will never have an effective battle against AIDS in Los Angeles," said Michael Weinstein, president of the AIDS Hospice Foundation; and the former head of the city-county Task Force on AIDS said that the county's response to AIDS has been characterized by an "egregious and shameful leadership vacuum." In 1989, Los Angeles County spent out of its own coffers only about 10 percent of what New York City spent on AIDS services; the total AIDS budget for the county, including state and federal funds, reached $60 million in 1989.

Nevertheless, the AIDS community is perhaps the one organized constituency in Los Angeles that has sufficient political clout to get a response to its demands from the conservative majority on the board of supervisors, providing a fascinating lesson in the value of organized political advocacy by a special population group that includes relatively affluent, politically active members. In the late 1980s, after organized, sustained, and highly visible political protests by AIDS groups and their behind-the-scenes political allies, the county board of supervisors voted to open a new AIDS hospice and to renovate completely an AIDS ward at LAC/USC Medical Center. The latter effort, undertaken against the recommendation of the Department of Health Services and using funds and round-the-clock work crews drawn from other building needs, in six months turned a single ward in the antiquated, half-century old facility into a modern and comfortable department, a match for almost any private hospital and a sharp contrast to all other departments at LAC/USC.

As with the rest of the health care system, insurance status determines where people with AIDS get care—from private or public physicians, clinics, and hospitals. In 1987, 81 percent of AIDS patient days in DHS facilities were covered by Medi-Cal, whereas 67 percent of AIDS patient days in Los Angeles private hospitals were reimbursed by private insurance and only 15 percent by Medi-Cal. In that year, DHS hospitals had 33 percent of all AIDS discharges in the county. As with its entire health care system, DHS does not have enough resources to meet the need for AIDS care. When a twenty-bed AIDS unit at LAC/USC Medical Center was opened in September 1989, it was immediately filled to capacity. Waits for an appointment at county outpatient AIDS clinics run as long as eight weeks. Los Angeles also lacks nursing home beds for AIDS patients. In the late 1980s, only 100 beds in residential nursing facilities were available for AIDS patients, and most of these were not state licensed and are therefore closed to Medi-Cal and other publicly funded patients.

Communicable Diseases and Immunization. Even in the area of public health services—the traditional responsibility of local health departments—funding and management of Los Angeles County's programs have been generally poor. According to Dr. Shirley Fanin, head of the county's communicable disease control programs, public health takes a back seat to medical care in the Los Angeles County DHS. Literally 90 percent of the more than $2 billion department budget goes to the hospitals, and more than a third of the remainder goes to five comprehensive health centers. Outside the hospitals, "priority" goes to staffing the health centers, so that field work and home visits are now "secondary."

Low funding and a variety of social factors have plagued county public health efforts to combat communicable diseases. TB rates, for example, are not dropping due in large part to high levels of immigration from Latin America and Southeast Asia.

Sexually transmitted disease rates have been rising. Although gonorrhea rates in Los Angeles are higher than for the country as a whole (509/100,000 population in Los Angeles; 312/100,000 in the United States), they declined 26 percent from 1986 to 1987. This improvement is probably due to changing sexual practices among male homosexuals and/or to a change in the strain of gonorrhea. The rate of penicillinase-producing neisserial gonorrhea (PPNG) has been going up, with almost all of the increase occurring among blacks. There has been an alarming increase of primary and secondary syphilis since 1984, also mostly among blacks, and by the late 1980s Los Angeles had a rate that was almost four times the national average (56/100,000 in Los Angeles, compared to 15/100,000 in the United States). According to Dr. Fanin, some forms of syphilis are "out of control." The increase in infectious syphilis has been attributed to a number of factors: reductions in public funding, a shifting of personnel to the AIDS prevention effort, the practice of exchanging sex for drugs, and the county's 1986 policy of charging $20 for an STD visit. Following a sharp decline in the number of clinic visits and an increase in the number of cases of syphilis, the county suspended the fees.

California law requires all children entering elementary school to be immunized against a range of communicable diseases. The county has done a good job over the last decade in working to ensure that children are adequately immunized. In 1979, 28.2 percent of children entering kindergarten needed one or more immunizations; by 1987, this number had decreased to 11.3 percent. Unfortunately, despite this increase in childhood immunizations, many poor and minority children remain inadequately protected against preventable diseases. Since late 1987, a rubeola (measles) epidemic has swept southern California, primarily affecting the prekindergarten children of poor Latino and black families. In January 1990 alone, Los Angeles County reported 260 suspected cases of measles.

Statewide, more than a third of the measles cases have required hospitalization, and by early 1990 the epidemic had killed twenty people.

In Los Angeles, as throughout the nation, local government provides a residual health system, the "provider of last resort." It serves the uninsured low-income population and the difficult, unprofitable cases that the private sector avoids. Its clientele are, for the most part, the poor and the powerless, and the care they receive tends to reflect their station in society. Despite its $2 billion budget and more than 23,000 staff positions, the Los Angeles County Department of Health Services remains woefully underfunded and understaffed. Although it logs 1 million inpatient days, 3 million outpatient visits, and 400,000 emergency room visits each year, the department cannot begin to meet the health problems and needs of Los Angeles' large and growing low-income population.

Competition Among Providers

"Competition is for survival."
—A Los Angeles Hospital CEO, December 2, 1988

"Virtually everything that can cause turbulence in a health-care environment is present in L.A."
—Paul Teslow, President and CEO, UniHealth America

The health care market in Los Angeles is highly competitive, as it has been for more than a century. Hospitals compete among themselves for privately insured patients, for physician loyalty, for nurses, and for HMO and PPO contracts. Physicians and hospitals also compete with each other, as do insurers, HMOs, and PPOs, all for their niche in the private market. Hospital administrators in Los Angeles describe the new competition as "tremendous," "vicious," and "horrendous."

This degree of competition did not exist in the early 1980s. Then, hospital administrators engaged in "bragging matches," telling one another about their most recent equipment acquisitions and about new administrative innovations. By the late 1980s, CEOs had become very guarded. They do not talk freely, commented one Westside CEO, "for fear you might give your competitor an idea or they may use what you tell them to take business away." Another CEO complained, "We used to have cooperation and sharing and now we [hospital administrators] can't get on the phone and talk." This CEO recently called a neighboring hospital to ask how its joint venture was organized and was told that the information would cost $3,000 in consulting fees.

Hospitals: Competition for and with Physicians

Hospitals are very dependent on physicians, especially those with large practices. For example, the "war" between two neighboring Los Angeles hospitals for the services of a successful heart specialist in 1986 was so intense that it made headlines in the *Los Angeles Times*. Contracts with medical groups are similarly prized. One hospital that emphasizes general acute care (rather than tertiary care services) gets fully half of its business from two medical groups—a family practice group and an internal medicine group.

Community hospitals have long competed for physicians by offering the latest pieces of equipment. However, hospital administrators interviewed for this study reported a new intensity in the competition for physicians. Hospitals woo physicians' staffs along with the physicians. In some tight competitive markets, hospital marketing representatives canvass community physicians monthly, providing information about the hospital's services. Some hospitals hold luncheons for the private office staffs of area physicians every three or six months. One hospital CEO described how, during these luncheons, hospital department heads are "paraded" out to sell the hospital. An American Medical International (AMI) hospital held one of these luncheons in its new staff dining room and offered lobster, steak, and crab salads, prepared by a Beverly Hills restaurant chef, along with new capital expenditures to encourage physician allegiance. This hospital also has a tuxedoed steward serve juice and coffee to its patients each morning, reminiscent of the efforts by hospitals at the turn of the century to attract paying patients.

The large teaching hospitals in Los Angeles are also part of the competitive environment. UCLA, for example, recently completed a large outpatient medical complex and physician office building, which it built so that it could keep its community-based physicians and, through them, the hospital's private patient base. "UCLA is in the game," said one Westside CEO. USC School of Medicine is also hoping to improve its academic and market position through the construction of a 275-bed seven story USC university hospital sponsored by National Medical Enterprises (NME). This hospital, which opened in 1991 in the middle of an economically deprived area, will be used by the medical school staff for private-pay patients only.

Hospitals compete with doctors as well as for them. Hospital and physician relations are, according to one CEO, a mix of "competition and cooperation. It's the damnedest love-hate relationship I ever knew." In Los Angeles, physicians are increasingly competing with hospitals in the provision of outpatient ancillary services; they are establishing their own vascular labs, imaging centers, outpatient surgi-centers, and other high-tech outpatient services.

Competition for HMO and PPO Contracts

If anything, hospital competition for HMO and PPO contracts is even more intense than is the competition for physicians. Without HMO and

PPO contracts, private Los Angeles hospitals, which run at about 50 percent occupancy, cannot survive. These contracts constitute a critical patient base: HMO and PPO contracts make up 20–25 percent of one downtown hospital's patient load; 17–20 percent at another; and 25 percent at one Westside hospital.

The percent of patients who belong to HMOs/PPOs is growing rapidly. For example, in 1987, AMI Tarzana Hospital, located in the San Fernando Valley of Los Angeles, had thirty managed-care contracts with insurance companies, employers, PPOs, and HMOs, representing about 20 percent of its gross revenues. By 1989, the hospital had fifty contracts, which accounted for 30 percent of its gross revenues.

The introduction of PPO (and Medi-Cal) contracting in the early 1980s found Los Angeles hospitals ill-prepared: Hospitals had to bid on an all-inclusive price but "How could we know what the price should be?" commented one CEO. Hospitals had "no information" upon which to make informed decisions. "It was a case of the blind leading the blind. Some of the early contracts were awful."

Hospital administrators have become more cautious in negotiating and monitoring contracts. UCLA Medical Center has about sixty managed-care contracts and will often spend five or six months negotiating a large contract. The number of HMO/PPO contracts differs by hospital and many contracts are inactive. One hospital CEO reported forty-eight PPO and four HMO contracts; another nearby hospital has ninety-five contracts. A downtown hospital administrator said his hospital has more than seventy-five contracts, of which only about two thirds are active, and a second downtown hospital CEO reported that only twenty to twenty-five of his hospital's 100 contracts were active. So many contracts add substantial administrative costs. One hospital has an elaborate preadmission review for all patients that is designed to screen for medical necessity and insurance coverage.

Competition for Nurses and Other Hospital Personnel

The Hospital Council of Southern California estimates that there are 5,000 unfilled nursing positions in Los Angeles. "It's a gas war out there," one nursing supervisor at a large Los Angeles hospital said of the competitive market. "Everyone has a problem" with nursing shortages, complained one CEO. To deal with this shortage and remain competitive, hospitals are increasing nursing salaries by as much as 20 percent or more a year. A 1988 study by the Hospital Council of Southern California found that the average starting pay for a bedside nurse who had just graduated from a two-year nursing program was $27,872 a year and that the average salary for a critical-care nurse who had received on-the-job training was $35,380. That year, hospital nursing salaries increased an average of 10.1 percent.

Not only do hospitals compete with one another for nurses, they also compete with the burgeoning number of registries that attract nurses by offering higher pay and greater flexibility. Thus, hospital nursing costs have skyrocketed because of the rising salaries and because of the increased reliance on registry nurses, which one CEO reported costs 2.5–3 times more than employing his own nurses. UCLA Medical Center, for example, spent $2.4 million for registry nurses in the last nine months of FY 1986-87. In the next fiscal year, the hospital spent nearly triple this amount, $6.1 million. Los Angeles County's six public hospitals spent $1 million for registry nurses in FY 1986-87, and the county projected that it would spend $12 million in FY 1988-89. In 1989, a Los Angeles public hospital paid $573.50 for a registry nurse to work a single twelve-hour weekend shift in critical care.

From the standpoint of nurses, registries seem advantageous; they provide more pay with greater flexibility. Hospitals, however, find that their dependence on registries is costly and that it compromises the continuity of care. Nurses who rotate through a hospital have little time to learn the hospital's routines or the special needs of individual patients.

To meet the nursing shortage and reduce their dependence on private registries, Los Angeles hospitals are trying a variety of internal strategies. CEOs, for example, are making greater use of nurse extenders, emergency medical technicians, and other support personnel to increase nurse productivity. After finding that nurses were spending only 30 percent of their time on patient care, one CEO transferred some nonpatient-care nursing duties to other staff in hopes of increasing nurses' direct patient-care time to 40–50 percent. If the nursing shortage is difficult for private Los Angeles hospitals, it is a true emergency for the county's public facilities, which are often forced to close beds temporarily because of inadequate staffing.

The Impact of Hospital Competition on Reimbursement

The 1980s were hard on Los Angeles hospitals. During the decade, hospitals confronted a new competitive environment in which private insurers, HMOs, and PPOs demanded and received discounted rates, in which Medicare and Medi-Cal substantially reduced reimbursement rates over previous levels, and in which the large and growing uninsured population placed new strains on emergency and inpatient finances.

The Move from Indemnity to PPO/HMO Contracts. Insurers and employers, confronted with continuing double-digit hospital inflation, responded almost immediately to the 1982 reform legislation by contracting prospectively for hospital rates. As PPO/HMO contracts proliferated, the number of patients covered by indemnity policies declined substantially. Indemnity contracts have almost become a thing of the past, according to Los Angeles hospital CEOs. At one hospital surveyed, 15 percent of the patients were covered by indemnity policies, but at three others, indemnity patients made up less than 10 percent of the census. With the decline in indemnity coverage, hospitals lost the ability to shift the cost of caring for uninsured patients onto privately insured patients.

Exact dollar figures on HMO/PPO contracts are not available. According to CEOs interviewed for this study, PPOs and HMOs receive sizeable discounts—18–50 percent off hospital charges. The director of the Hospital Council of Southern California commented that contracts are a "nightmare for hospitals." Besides incurring the administrative costs of handling fifty to one hundred contracts, hospitals often do not get fair prices for their contracts, he noted. If a PPO constitutes only 2–3 percent of a hospital's business, the hospital will contract to cover "marginal costs," he explained. However, if the patient mix changes and the PPO begins to make up 15 percent of the hospital's business, the hospital "can be in trouble."

Serious negotiations occur before contracts are signed. Yet, even after six years' experience with contracting, hospital administrators admitted to a randomness in the negotiating process. Two contracts providing the same services to similar populations can vary significantly in price. One CEO likened the contracting process to "buying a car," where incentives are offered, such as "AM-FM stereo and whitewalls," in order to get a better price. He has told PPOs with which he was negotiating that if they will agree to a higher price, he would, for example, "throw in smoking prevention and weight-loss programs."

PPOs and HMOs promise to increase the patient loads of hospitals in return for the negotiated discount. If contracts are inactive or if they do not increase volume, they are discontinued. Whereas some contracts do not increase volume, others have proved beneficial. One hospital administrator reported that a Blue Shield contract resulted in an increase in his hospital's market area and its patient volume. When interviewed he was "trying like hell" to get a Blue Cross contract as well. However, he said that insurers will often limit the number of hospitals in a community with which they contract because they must assure hospitals of a sufficient volume to get reduced rates. The deal is "a discount from the hospital in return for more patients."

According to another CEO, HMOs and PPOs play "hospitals against each other by going to a nearby facility if they don't get the discount they want from a particular hospital." This administrator said that HMOs and PPOs, despite their claims to be concerned with quality, are interested only in the discount.

Reimbursement methods for managed-care contracts vary. For some contracts, hospitals receive a flat per diem, giving them an incentive to hold down intensity. More commonly, hospitals are paid a percentage of a capitation payment, giving them an incentive to hold down admissions.

Some CEOs said they prefer capitation arrangements because they are more profitable than per diem contracts.

Medi-Cal Selective Contracting. Promising hospitals greater volume for discounted per diem reimbursement rates, California contracted with a total of 109 Los Angeles hospitals between April 1983 and December 1989 to provide care to Medi-Cal patients. Contracting hospitals have not fared well. Contracts are secret, and thus the exact amount of reimbursement for each hospital is not known. However, in the first few years of contracting, a large number of hospitals complained that they received no increases in their per diem reimbursement rate. Statewide, from 1984 through 1988, the average contract rate increased 10.3 percent, an average of 2.6 percent per year. In 1989, the state was more generous, increasing statewide rates by an average of 4. 0 percent.

In California, inflation-adjusted contractual allowances (the difference between charges and the amount actually paid) for Medi-Cal, which were $431 million (4.4 percent of revenue) in 1981-82, increased 123 percent by 1985-86 (to 6.4 percent of revenue). County teaching and nonteaching hospitals incurred the greatest burden of unreimbursed costs due to Medi-Cal, at 8.8 percent and 9.5 percent of revenues, respectively, in 1985-86. But, private and University of California teaching hospitals were close behind, at 8.6 percent of revenue. According to data provided by the Hospital Council of Southern California, in the first quarter of 1988, Medi-Cal patients accounted for 19 percent of discharges but only 11 percent of revenues. In 1988, Medi-Cal paid an average per diem to southern California hospitals of $567 (up from $516 in 1984), an amount a Hospital Council representative said covered only 60–70 percent of the costs of care. Los Angeles hospitals reported that during the last quarter of 1987 and the first three quarters of 1988, they incurred $954.3 million in Medi-Cal contractual adjustments, up 25.5 percent from the previous four quarters.

Low reimbursement rates have led some hospitals to terminate their Medi-Cal contracts. At the end of 1989, because of contract terminations, hospital closures, and facility conversions, the number of contracting hospitals serving the Medi-Cal population was 30 percent less than in 1983. In 1988 and 1989 alone, fifteen Los Angeles hospitals terminated their contracts. Of these, three closed, one became a chemical-dependency hospital, and one recontracted at the end of 1989. The remaining ten no longer serve Medi-Cal patients. In one Los Angeles community, four of the five Medi-Cal hospital providers terminated their contracts, forcing the state to open the area to fee-for-service reimbursement.

It may be that the years of tight Medi-Cal reimbursement budgets are over. Fearful that some hospitals with large Medi-Cal patient loads would drop out of the system, the State Department of Health Services began providing extra contract funding in 1987. Two downtown hospitals with

Medi-Cal contracts that have been suffering large deficits due to serving uninsured patients and low Medi-Cal reimbursements reported that Medi-Cal improved their contracted per diem rates. One of these hospitals received two separate increases, totaling 10 percent, in its per diem in 1987 and early 1988 and then requested and received another increase in the latter half of 1988. These "significant" increases were justified, said the hospital's CEO, because of the hospital's heavy obstetrics load, its substantial, disproportional share of Medi-Cal patients, and its emergency room losses. Medi-Cal, he believes, is responding more favorably to the needs of contracting hospitals than it was a few years ago because of "the threat of some major hospitals going under. " To obtain increases in their rates, the CEO believes, hospitals must be able to put political pressure on Medi-Cal or have good, justifiable reasons for the increases. In the case of his hospital, "We had both."

Studies have found that selective contracting saved the state millions of dollars, especially in the early years of implementation, and did not decrease access to inpatient hospital care for the poor. For the most part, hospitals that bid in good faith for contracts were those that already carried the heaviest Medi-Cal loads.

If selective contracting did not diminish access to care for the Medi-Cal population, it did further segregate in separate hospitals the Medi-Cal and uninsured populations from privately insured and Medicare patients. A large number of hospitals in advantageous financial positions, like Cedars-Sinai, chose not to contract. "A Medi-Cal contract has become a symbol of a certain kind of hospital," said Lucien Wulsin, chief staff consultant for the Assembly Special Committee on Medi-Cal Oversight. Contracting allowed the "suburban facilities to walk away from any responsibility for the poor."

Medicare Reimbursement. Still adjusting to the competitive 1982 reforms, the hospital industry was in poor shape to deal with the federal government's 1984 Medicare prospective payment system (PPS). PPS was especially traumatic for California hospitals for two reasons. First, patients in California hospitals had a lower average length of stay (ALOS) than the national average. In 1983, the ALOS was 6.4 days in California, compared to 7.6 days nationwide. Thus, hospitals in California had less leeway than hospitals elsewhere to reap the early benefits of PPS through a substantial reduction in inpatient days per DRG. Second, the state's hospitals are some of the most expensive in the nation. In 1983, total expenses per patient day in California were $662, compared to $426 for all hospitals nationwide; hospital expenses per admission were $4,267 in California, compared to $3,221 nationwide. The slow move to a national PPS rate meant that California hospitals lost out financially to hospitals in other states where costs were below the national average.

As in all communities, hospitals in Los Angeles depend on Medicare patients for survival. In the first quarter of 1988, Medicare patients in Los Angeles hospitals represented 28 percent of discharges and 32 percent of revenues. Administrators in those hospitals argue that Medicare's PPS does not pay adequately to cover costs. Analysis of state data does indicate that Medicare reimbursement has been reduced. Medicare inflation-adjusted contractual allowances for all California hospitals, which were $1 billion (8.8 percent of revenue) in 1981-82, increased 60 percent by 1985-86 (to 10. 7 percent of revenue). For the four quarters ending September 30, 1988, Los Angeles acute care hospitals reported $1.59 billion dollars in Medicare contractual allowances.

Uncompensated Care. The health care needs of Los Angeles County's 2.1 million uninsured residents put a financial burden on the county's private hospitals. Loss of the ability to cost-shift and the continuing need for capital expenditures make these uncompensated-care costs difficult to absorb.

A study by Lewin and Associates found that the state's private hospitals provide less charity care than similar institutions in four other states (Florida, North Carolina, Tennessee, and Virginia). The study found that uncompensated care (defined as charity care and bad debt) accounted for about 3 percent of expenses for California's private hospitals in 1985 and 1986, compared with up to 10 percent in the four other states studied. Moreover, the study found that nonprofit hospitals in the four other study states provided 50 percent to 120 percent more uncompensated care than for-profit institutions, whereas in California the difference was only 15 percent. The lower uncompensated-care burden among California's private hospitals is undoubtedly due to the still extensive network of county hospitals that absorb much of the load.

Uncompensated-care costs in the state and in the county grew throughout the 1980s. In FY 1985-86, California hospitals provided almost a billion dollars ($975 million) in uncompensated care to uninsured patients—84 percent more than in 1981-82 (49 percent more after adjusting for inflation). Almost half of this amount ($468 million) was provided by the state's network of public county hospitals; private hospitals provided the remaining $507 million.

Los Angeles hospitals reported spending over $866.7 million in bad debt and charity care for the four quarters ending September 30, 1988. This uncompensated care load was not spread evenly among hospitals. While some hospitals provide little uncompensated care, others do more than their share. A study by the *Los Angeles Times* found that in FY 1986-87, 40 of the 127 community hospitals in Los Angeles County provided 90 percent of the uncompensated care. Of these 40 hospitals, 26 had uncompensated-care burdens of less than 5 percent of expenses. Hospitals in Los Angeles County expended a total of $371 million in uncompensated care during FY 1986-87, 59.7 percent of which was provided by the five public county hospitals. During the 1980s, with the growth of the uninsured population, a number of Los Angeles hospitals found that uncompensated care threatened their continued survival.

The Impact of Competition on Hospital Survival

Faced with the problems of growing uncompensated care, increased competition, a heavy debt burden, and lower reimbursement rates, sixteen hospitals in Los Angeles County closed their doors between 1980 and 1989. Four other hospitals converted from acute-care to specialty facilities, one hospital became a skilled nursing facility (SNF), and another, an outpatient clinic. In 1989 only one hospital closed, merging with a neighboring institution that had already missed more than one payment on its capital debt; both hospitals served Medi-Cal and low-income uninsured patients. Others, however, are in financial difficulty. In 1989, a Chinatown hospital, straining under a combined Medicare and Medi-Cal patient load of 85–90 percent, declared bankruptcy, and San Pedro Peninsula Hospital confirmed that it was in technical default on an $18 million bond issue. In early 1990, another hospital announced plans to declare bankruptcy. The president of the Hospital Council of Southern California predicted that about nine or ten more hospitals in Los Angeles would close by 1992.

The decade of the 1980s was especially difficult for the for-profit hospitals in Los Angeles, many of which belong to large for-profit chains headquartered in Los Angeles. The very characteristics of for-profit hospitals that allowed them to prosper in the cost-based reimbursement era of the 1970s and early 1980s, such as patients' short length of stay and substantial mark-up on ancillary services, undermined their financial health when the reimbursement system changed. Although for-profit hospitals, like their not-for-profit brethren, did well in the first part of the decade, their fortunes plummeted in early 1986 when Medicare began serious efforts to lower reimbursement rates and made other changes in the system. National Medical Enterprises (NME), for example, realized an additional $25 million from Medicare in the first year after PPS was introduced. But, according to Donald Thayer, vice president for development at the corporation, the Medicare party ended quickly. The combination of the adjustment of capital reimbursement, the loss of return on equity, and the blending of hospital-specific to national rates led to a decrease of $30 million in revenues for the firm the following year. In the first three months of 1986, the Los Angeles–based firm posted its first quarterly loss ever and announced that it would sell nine hospitals. In the second quarter of that year, American Medical International (AMI), another for-profit chain based in Los Angeles, recorded a loss of $82 million, its first red ink ever.

At the start of the 1990s, many Los Angeles hospitals found themselves in a precarious financial condition. The Hospital Council of Southern California reported that half of all Los Angeles County hospitals were running in the red. Yet, a report by Baltimore-based Health Care Investment Analysts showed that Los Angeles hospitals were slightly more profitable than hospitals nationally, posting an average operating margin of 0.39 percent, compared to 0.22 percent for all U.S. hospitals.

Moreover, a number of Los Angeles hospitals believe they have turned the financial corner. The hospital CEOs interviewed for this study all thought that their hospitals had weathered the storm. Los Angeles hospitals that made it through the 1980s adopted a number of survival strategies, as discussed in the following sections.

Responding to New Reimbursement Incentives

The change from cost-based reimbursement to flat DRG Medicare payments, flat per diem Medi-Cal rates, and discount rates paid under PPO and HMO contracts imposed new incentives for hospitals to cut inpatient days. Although ALOS in Los Angeles hospitals was generally lower than elsewhere, the hospitals found the new PPS to be a great enough incentive to cut Medicare inpatient days further. Though physicians did not want hospitals to dictate how they should practice medicine, reported one CEO, reducing the length of stay was "a matter of survival" for the institutions. This CEO showed each physician the discrepancy between, say, the $100,000 in costs generated by that physician and the $35, 000 in reimbursements related to those costs. The hospital also eliminated standing orders that required seven tests (including chest x-rays) for all new admissions and leveraged cooperation from doctors by promising them new equipment, such as an imaging center, if the profit margin improved.

Steve Gamble, president of the Hospital Council of Southern California, reported that physicians clearly changed their practice patterns as a result of PPS. Hospital CEOs pushed physicians to reduce the length of stay for Medicare patients, he said, but were then "surprised" when physicians changed their practice for all patients.

The change in practice patterns for privately insured patients was probably more the result of pressure from insurers than the result of the physicians' general acceptance of the new order. Nurses employed by Prudential Insurance Company, for example, visit 80 percent of their plan's Los Angeles inpatients to check on their status and readiness for discharge.

Hospital efforts to reduce length of stay were successful. One Westside hospital reported that the hospital's nine to ten day average length of stay in 1983 had fallen to 5.6 days by 1988. Similarly, ALOS for Medicare patients at that hospital was cut by over five days, from fourteen to sixteen days in 1984 to about eight days in 1988. Within the county as a whole,

ALOS for acute-care beds dropped from 6.6 in 1981 to 6. 0 in 1987. Medicare inpatients in Los Angeles stay in the hospital an average of 8.17 days.

By 1987, the drive to reduce length of stay had taken its toll on hospital occupancy rates. Throughout the county, the average occupancy rate for general acute-care beds dropped from 58.1 percent in 1981 to 51.7 percent in 1987. In the nation as a whole, the average occupancy rate in 1987 was 60 percent. Faced with a dramatic reduction in inpatient days and revenue, hospitals were forced to look for other ways to increase their bottom line.

Moving from Inpatient to Outpatient Care. As the federal government and private insurers tightened up inpatient reimbursement, hospitals responded by moving patients to the less regulated, less controlled, and thus more profitable outpatient department. Hospital and insurance executives interviewed for this study all commented about the radical change in the way hospitals operate. Whatever procedures and tests could be moved to the outpatient department were moved; diagnostic and surgical procedures for such conditions as ectopic pregnancies, that formerly required lengthy inpatient admissions, are now routinely done in the outpatient departments of all major Los Angeles hospitals.

The number of outpatient surgeries performed in Los Angeles hospitals increased dramatically: By 1987, 44.7 percent of all hospital surgeries were performed in outpatient departments, compared to 18 percent in 1981. The amount of revenue generated by hospital outpatient departments increased steadily along with the number of procedures performed. At one downtown hospital, outpatient care, which accounted for 15 percent of revenues in 1985 and 1986, increased to about 25 percent of revenues in 1988.

Joining Together with Other Hospitals. For many Los Angeles hospitals, belonging to or joining multihospital systems enabled them to stay afloat during the turbulent 1980s. Although for-profit hospital chains reduced their hospital holdings, chain membership proved critical to the survival of many not-for-profit hospitals. The CEO of one Lutheran hospital stated that he was "fairly positive that the hospital would not have continued" in the face of heavy operating losses without the backup of the Lutheran Hospital Society, which helped the hospital refinance its debt at 1 to 1.5 points less than it had been paying and covered some of its operating deficit.

In June 1989, the Lutheran Hospital Society and Health West merged to form UniHealth America, doubling the size of each of the organizations. This merger, said another Lutheran hospital CEO, helped his hospital in two ways. First, it put the fourteen hospitals in the system in a better position to contract with areawide PPOs and HMOs because they could provide hospital services in a large area of southern California. Second, the merger significantly helped the CEO's hospital with debt financing, allowing the hospital to refinance its outstanding debt from a 9.25 percent to a 7.5 percent interest rate.

The CEO of a Catholic hospital felt as positive as the Lutheran hospital CEO about the benefits of chain membership, although his hospital was the chain's only facility in southern California. According to the CEO, chain membership helps with "purchasing, legal counsel, and debt financing."

Nonprofit "free-standing" hospitals are also joining together for survival. For example, in a notable 1988 merger, Queen of Angels Hospital closed and merged with the newly rebuilt but debt-ridden Hollywood Presbyterian Hospital. The hospitals were operating at 40 percent and 45 percent occupancy rates, respectively. The merger, said the chairman of the trust that owns Hollywood Presbyterian, is "a sign of the times. We're just the first." This prediction was echoed by other hospital CEOs interviewed for this study. With the exception of a few hospitals, such as Cedars-Sinai, "stand-alone" hospitals would become extinct, "like dinosaurs," predicted one CEO.

Caution with Regard to Capital Expenditures and Joint Ventures with Physicians. Los Angeles hospitals have become more cautious about large capital expenditures. Hospital administrators described how they had become "more careful" about capital decisions and were quick to point out that a number of hospitals in financial trouble in the 1980s, like Hollywood Presbyterian, had undertaken major modernization or rebuilding projects for which they could not service their debt.

Yet, this new caution notwithstanding, Los Angeles hospitals, spurred by competition, have continued to expend large sums of money on capital equipment and buildings. During the 1980s, hospitals continued to upgrade equipment and remodel their physical plants and were venturing outside the hospital, often in collaboration with physicians, to find new market opportunities.

The state's virtual elimination of health planning legislation during the 1980s made it easy for hospitals in California to remodel existing physical plants and purchase expensive new equipment. In 1983 and 1984, the legislature significantly weakened the state's health planning law, and in 1986, the law was repealed altogether. In the four quarters ending March 31, 1989, Los Angeles County's 164 acute-care hospitals spent over $500 million on capital, 25. 6 percent more money than they had spent in the previous four quarters. Continued capital expenditures resulted in fiscal problems for a number of hospitals that had difficulty servicing their debt burdens.

Competition does not seem to have affected the excess growth of hospital specialty services in California or in Los Angeles. Indeed, as one California policy analyst suggested, the 1982 reforms may have promoted "service expansion so that a hospital appears as 'full service' to potential contractors." From 1981 through 1987, the number of Los Angeles hospitals performing cardiovascular surgeries increased from thirty-three to thirty-eight, and the number performing cardiac catheterizations went from forty-seven to fifty.

Hospital capital expenditures were made not just for modernization and new equipment but also for the establishment of speciality services within hospitals, such as skilled nursing home beds and psychiatric or drug/alcohol treatment wings. At least two acute-care Los Angeles hospitals converted not only beds but their entire facilities—one became a chemical dependency hospital, and the other became an acute psychiatric hospital.

With the exception of the new NME/USC Medical School hospital, no new general acute-care hospital began construction or opened its doors during the 1980s (although a number of existing hospitals were totally rebuilt). However, free-standing specialty hospitals or "boutiques," often built by for-profit chains, were faddish in the decade: A new eye hospital, an Alzheimer's hospital, several facilities designed for people to recuperate from plastic surgery, as well as a number of alcohol/drug-treatment facilities opened in Los Angeles. These hospitals cater to the rich. For example, Midway Hospital's cosmetic surgery postoperative recuperation facility, called "Entretemps," charges $225 a night for a "postoperative sojourn" in its "luxurious recuperative retreat." The facility has private suites, chauffeur services to and from physicians' offices, and twenty-four-hour nursing care.

Although the new reimbursement system of the 1980s strained hospital-physician relations as never before, it also led to new ventures in financial cooperation between hospitals and their physicians. In the second half of the decade, Los Angeles hospitals and physicians began a large number of for-profit joint ventures in a wide range of services, including imaging centers, radiology, free-standing outpatient clinics, physical therapy, and medical office buildings.

Not-for-profit as well as for-profit hospitals adopted the joint venture strategy. Generally, nonprofit hospitals set up for-profit subsidiaries with physicians as limited partners. For example, one Westside voluntary hospital established a joint venture imaging center with eighty physicians. In 1988, a year and a half after the center opened, it began making a profit, which is shared by the hospital and investing physicians in proportion to their investment. A nearby hospital formed a joint venture with its physicians to build the hospital's office building; it also opened a joint venture free-standing ambulatory care/surgi-center in Beverly Hills and is considering additional joint ventures to provide MRI and lithotripsy services.

Like early HMO/PPO contracts, joint ventures were at first "put together in haste" and did not produce the kind of volume and revenues hospitals were hoping for. Now, hospitals and physicians reportedly look at joint ventures as purely business deals, assessing their value in terms of profits that can be realized rather than in terms of hoped-for volume.

Caution concerning joint ventures does not seem to apply to National Medical Enterprises, which establishes entire facilities as joint ventures "to provide incentives for doctors to practice there." An NME executive said that the firm relies "on the entrepreneurial drive of doctors" and knows that its joint ventures verge "on fraud and abuse, which is buying patients or paying doctors to bring them in." Although NME claims to avoid this, it provides very attractive terms for its physician partners.

Philanthropy. As profit margins declined during the 1980s, Los Angeles nonprofit hospitals rediscovered philanthropy. Philanthropy has "come full circle," explained one CEO. Fund raising has been especially important for capital improvements. The $31 million raised by one Westside hospital has been "significant," commented a CEO, and is one of the reasons the hospital has no capital debt. A number of Los Angeles hospitals have found movie stars, often through providing them care, to be particularly helpful in their fund-raising drives. Celebrity golf tournaments, relay marathons, and other events sponsored by movie stars raise millions of dollars for the community's hospitals. The most successful hospital fund raiser, held by 1,108-bed Cedars-Sinai Medical Center, raised $90 million in the past few years.

Reducing Uncompensated Care: Impact on Access

Unlike a number of other states, California does not have a system for reimbursing hospitals that provide a disproportionate amount of charity care. Los Angeles hospitals, without coverage for their uninsured patients and having to deal with fewer paying inpatients, lower reimbursement rates and profit margins, and large capital debt burdens, adopted a number of strategies to reduce their uninsured patient load. Most prominently, they eliminated services that resulted in high uncompensated-care costs. For example, because so many burn victims are uninsured, a number of hospitals in the late 1980s reduced or eliminated their intensive care burn units. In 1989, the county's remaining three burn centers had a total of twelve staffed intensive care beds, down from thirty-four in 1987. Burn patients regularly must be flown hundreds of miles to hospitals in other parts of California and even in neighboring states because empty beds cannot be found for them in Los Angeles.

Some private hospitals are also becoming more unwilling to serve the poor. For example, the NME/USC Medical School hospital, which was built in one of the poorest communities in Los Angeles to accommodate the private patients of medical school faculty, will not offer emergency, maternity, or pediatric services nor will it provide care to Medi-Cal patients. USC argues that the hospital will increase faculty attendance at LAC/USC Medical Center, but most observers are skeptical of that argument. UCLA Medical Center has also limited the number of Medi-Cal patients it will see in its adult general medicine clinic, a sore point for some faculty who believe the state-supported University of California hospital should serve all patients in the state program.

Emergency Care Gridlock. For the same reason that burn beds have been eliminated, hospitals have drastically reduced the county's capacity to handle emergency and trauma patients. Under both state and federal law, hospitals with emergency rooms are required to stabilize all emergency room patients before transferring them and cannot transfer any patient without the consent of the receiving hospital.

Emergency rooms, then, are the one unlocked door by which the uninsured can obtain care in private hospitals. Once uninsured patients are in the hospital, CEOs report that it often is difficult to transfer them to public facilities because they are full. A 1987 one-month survey of most Los Angeles private and county hospitals with emergency rooms found that county hospitals treated 55.5 percent of all the uninsured emergency patients. Among the fifty-one private hospitals that provided care to the other 45.5 percent of emergency patients, fifteen with trauma centers treated almost as many of these patients as the other thirty-six private hospitals; these fifteen hospitals incurred $3.9 million in unreimbursed costs for emergency care in just this one month. As many as 25 percent of a hospital's emergency patients may be uninsured, according to the hospital CEOs interviewed for this study. One downtown hospital reported losses of $6 million a year in its emergency department; another reported losses of $3–$5 million a year.

Faced with mounting uncompensated-care costs associated with emergency rooms and trauma center operations, hospitals, starting in 1986, began closing these services. At least three emergency rooms have closed, and in January 1988, Methodist Hospital in the San Gabriel Valley, citing losses of $1.5 million a year, became the tenth private hospital to pull out of the four-year old trauma system. Of the original twenty-three trauma centers, only thirteen are left to serve the more than 8 million people in Los Angeles County.

Some observers believe that emergency room closures are the result of physician pressure on hospitals. Lucien Wulsin of the Assembly Special Committee on Medi-Cal Oversight commented that neurosurgeons were asking from $1,000 to $1,500 a day for staffing a trauma center. He claimed that physician demands are "what broke the bank. Hospitals don't want to get on their doctors because they don't want them to leave the hospital."

The hospitals that are still operating emergency rooms and trauma centers are overwhelmed with patients and repeatedly declare their emergency services closed, forcing paramedic units to travel further and further to find open emergency departments for critically ill patients. This situation occurs every day on a small scale, but several times a week as many as a dozen or more hospitals in central, south-central, and west Los Angeles have simultaneously shut their emergency room doors. For example, on March 1, 1989, thirty-four Los Angeles hospitals closed their ERs, some several times during the day. Said Alan Cowan, chief paramedic for the Los Angeles City Fire Department, "Our entire system has had a cardiac arrest."

Although many hospitals close their ERs temporarily because their ERs or their ICU beds are "saturated," Los Angeles County investigators found that some hospitals close their doors when they still have sufficient unused ER capacity. These hospitals—and others that have threatened to downgrade their emergency rooms and thus close them altogether to "911" rescue ambulances—are simply using this devise to reduce their indigent patient load.

The ER/trauma center crisis has received tremendous press coverage and has become a hot political issue because temporary and permanent closures pose a major peril to middle- and upper-income residents of Los Angeles. By the end of the 1980s, the medical care crisis afflicting the poor of Los Angeles had spilled over onto the rest of society, creating concern for the future of the entire health care delivery system.

Health Resources

Fierce competition for profits and the downward pressure on revenues have affected hospital, long-term-care facilities and services, physicians, and nurses.

Hospitals

As in the rest of the country, the number of community hospital beds per 1,000 Los Angeles residents and the number of Los Angeles community hospitals have been shrinking. The number of community hospitals fell from 144 in 1980 to 127 in 1987. In 1988, an additional hospital in Los Angeles closed. With this shrinking hospital capacity, the number of hospital beds declined from 4.33 per 1,000 population in 1980 to 3.75 per 1,000 in 1987.

Community hospitals in Los Angeles are dominated by not-for-profit facilities. Although the not-for-profits represented only 47 percent of all community hospitals in 1987, they accounted for 59 percent of all licensed beds. Investor-owned hospitals tend to be smaller than the nonprofit hospitals, have less sophisticated medical technology, and have lower occupancy rates, with the result that they have less impact on medical care in the county than their 50 percent share of the hospitals would suggest. Among investor-owned hospitals, hospital corporations play a significant role. In 1983, they owned 35.3 percent of all community hospitals in the county, compared to 15.4 percent for investor-owned independent hospitals, 14.0 percent for not-for-profit independent institutions, and 30.9 percent for not-for-profit chain hospitals.

For-profit facilities have increased their number and share of specialty hospitals by opening small facilities, resulting in a declining average number of beds. Most of these new specialty hospitals are private substance-abuse and psychiatric facilities. Excluding state hospitals, investor-owned hospitals increased their share of specialty hospital beds from 33 percent in 1980 to 36 percent in 1987, and not-for-profit hospitals decreased their share from 36 percent to 32 percent. Overall, specialty hospital beds declined from 1.25 per 1,000 population in 1980 to .88 per 1,000 in 1987.

Nursing Homes

The number of long-term-care beds in Los Angeles has not kept up with the aging of the population. In 1987-88, the county had 387 nursing homes, five fewer than it did in 1980-81. Although the number of beds increased slightly, this growth was outstripped by the growing elderly population. The number of nursing home beds per 100 persons aged sixty-five or over declined from 5.27 in 1980-81 to 4.94 in 1987-88. This lack of growth was the result of a number of factors, not the least of which was new competition from hospital SNF units, licensed as "distinct parts" (DPs) .

Nursing home care in Los Angeles is a for-profit enterprise. Between 1980 and 1987, the percent of long-term-care facilities owned by church and other nonprofit organizations decreased by about one-third, from 19 percent of the total to 13 percent. Long-term care facilities were sold to for-profit nursing home chains, which by the end of the decade owned 39 percent of the area's facilities, up from 17 percent in 1980.

Reimbursement, Costs, and Competition. The phase-out of California's health planning law did not lead to a flurry of nursing home construction, as it did in a number of other states. During the latter part of the 1980s, nursing homes lost much of their profitability. Although operating at over 90 percent occupancy, nursing home firms saw little financial advantage in building new facilities. According to Robert Van Tuyle, past CEO of Beverly Enterprises, low reimbursement rates, especially for Medi-Cal patients, make new homes unprofitable. Beverly Enterprises, the nation's largest nursing home chain, will not build a facility in California unless market research shows that it will have a minimum of 50 percent private-pay patients. Sometimes its requirement is for 70 percent private-pay patients. "We can't build and fill a facility with Medi-Cal patients and break even, " Van Tuyle said.

As with hospital care, Medi-Cal reimburses nursing homes less than other payers do. In Los Angeles County, Medi-Cal patients utilize 69 percent of all nursing home days but contribute only 60 percent of total net revenues. In 1988, Medicare and private-pay patients made up 3 percent and 28 percent of the nursing home population but accounted for 5 percent and 36 percent of nursing home revenues, respectively.

California Medi-Cal rates are below the rates paid by the Medicaid programs of other states. On average, Medi-Cal pays nursing homes about $10 less than the average Medicaid rate nationwide. However, state audits of nursing home reports do not entirely support the perception that nursing homes lose money on every Medi-Cal patient. A report by Lewin and Associates found that 54 percent of California nursing homes make profits on their Medi-Cal patients: "The [Medi-Cal] system as a whole is providing a net positive margin to the industry," the Lewin study found. Beverly Enterprises also made a profit on the vast majority of its ninety California nursing homes.

Increasing operating costs may also have dampened the enthusiasm for nursing home growth. The nursing shortage and a booming economy that led to a paucity of minimum-wage workers forced Los Angeles nursing homes to increase wages significantly.

The expansion of hospitals into the area of nursing home care also damaged profitability, complained Larry Hinman, representative from the California Association for Health Facilities. Starting about 1985, the larger acute care hospitals in the county set aside "distinct part" beds to care for nursing home patients. These beds are supposed to be for long-term-care patients who need slightly more intensive medical care than what is available in nursing homes, but according to Hinman, little oversight is exercised over the level of care needed by these patients. Many of these patients, Hinman believes, would be more appropriately placed in nursing homes.

Finally, the repeal of the Medicare catastrophic legislation hurt the nursing home industry, substantially reducing the number of Medicare nursing home patients. According to data from the California Association of Health Facilities, with Medicare's catastrophic nursing home benefit in effect, the percent of Los Angeles nursing home patients covered by Medicare jumped to 18 percent in 1989; by the end of January 1990, following the repeal of the legislation, this number had plummeted to 3–4 percent.

Because of low reimbursement rates, increasing wages, and, probably, poor business decisions, many nursing homes, like hospitals and insurers, faced rocky financial times in the latter part of the 1980s. Beverly Enterprises, for example, lost $30.5 million in 1987, $23.9 million in 1988, and approximately $103 million in 1989.

Access. Although private-pay nursing home patients and those covered by Medicare have no trouble finding nursing home beds, the same cannot be said for Medi-Cal beneficiaries. Medi-Cal patients take up a majority of all nursing home beds in the county, but they are not sought after. Given the reimbursement differential between Medi-Cal and other payers, nursing homes routinely give preference to private-pay and Medicare patients. Many Medi-Cal patients are initially admitted to nursing homes as private-pay patients, and only later convert to Medi-Cal after "spending down" their resources to qualify for the program.

For hospitals, finding reasonably located nursing home placements for their elderly poor patients is difficult, if not impossible. Said one Westside hospital discharge planner, "It is with great rarity that my co-workers and I are successful in placing these [Medi-Cal] patients locally." Another discharge planner called the lack of Medi-Cal beds a "human tragedy."

Although most nursing homes in Los Angeles are Medi-Cal certified, many will not accept new Medi-Cal patients. A study of nursing homes in the Santa Monica area, for instance, found that although fifteen of twenty-two nursing homes in the city of Santa Monica and the surrounding community were Medi-Cal certified, most refused to take new Medi-Cal patients.

Quality. On paper, California has a rigorous nursing home inspection program. In Los Angeles County, the Department of Health Services contracts with the state to inspect all nursing homes in the county on a yearly basis and to follow up all consumer complaints, often with surprise inspections. Yet, despite frequent inspections, quality-of-care problems continue to plague the state's nursing home industry.

The state's inspection system is a paper tiger, said a representative of a state watchdog agency, the Commission on California State Government Organization and Economy, commonly known as the Little Hoover Commission. Nursing homes rarely lose their licenses but instead are fined for violations of quality standards. However, fines have been ineffective in improving quality. A study of state citations by the *Los Angeles Times* reported that a nursing home found to have been the "direct proximate cause of a patient death" might be fined $15,000 to $25,000. A nursing home could be fined $10,000 if a patient has a bed sore that has reached the bone and requires surgery. Rapes lead to fines of $6,000 to $7,000; falsification of medical records might lead to a fine of $7,000.

Of the $5.3 million in fines levied against nursing home operators in 1985, about $2.1 million was forgiven when operators corrected deficiencies, and only $1.1 million was expected to be collected. Nursing homes can appeal citations almost indefinitely and delay paying fines.

Despite repeated violations of quality standards, nursing homes in the state make profits. Beverly Enterprises, which was fined $724,000 in 1986 and put on probation for gross quality-of-care violations, reported more than $14 million in before-tax profits from its California operations, although nationally the firm had a negative profit margin. In 1988, one of the chain's Los Angeles nursing homes, for example, made $241,000 in before-tax profits despite a citation that year for not providing "sufficient quantities of diapers, pillows, bed sheets and wash cloths to maintain patient care needs."

The Medi-Cal reimbursement system provides incentives for poor quality. A study by Lewin and Associates found that paying a per diem rate with little scrutiny on whether the money is spent on patient care results "in the state paying profits to some facilities that spend very little on nursing care for Medi-Cal patients."

Lack of scrutiny of physicians is another cause of poor quality of care. In 1989, the Little Hoover Commission issued a scathing report on physicians who provide substandard care to their nursing home patients. Michael Parks, former director of the Nursing Home Advocacy Project at Bet Tzedek Legal Services in Los Angeles, confirmed this assessment: "There's been an abdication of medical responsibility by physicians," he stated. "The vast majority of doctors won't go in a nursing home, and those that do are often considered lackeys of the home."

Home Health Agencies

At the start of 1986, 127 home health agencies (HHAs) were licensed to operate in Los Angeles County. Because a number of these agencies were not providing care or were delicensed later in 1986, only 111 home health agencies reported to the state that year. Members of these agencies visited over 93,000 patients, making more than 1.1 million visits during the year.

Home health agencies run the gamut in size and sponsorship from the nonprofit Visiting Nurses Association (VNA) to the chain-owned Upjohn and Kimberly agencies to small home health providers established by hospitals. Like nursing homes, home health agencies are disproportionately for-profit enterprises: 62 percent of home health agencies in Los Angeles are for-profit, and 39 percent are not-for-profit. The nonprofit HHAs are more likely to be owned by hospitals than their for-profit counterparts (46.7 percent, compared to 8.2 percent) and are significantly larger.

Growth and Competition. Home health agencies grew at a rapid rate during the early 1980s in response to changes in the federal Medicare law that eliminated the prior hospitalization requirement and the 100-visit limit. From 1971 through 1979, a total of 135 new home health agencies were licensed in the state; from 1980 through 1985, 365 new home health agencies began operations.

Beginning in the mid-1980s, however, this growth rate slowed as the smaller HHAs went out of business and consolidated. A number of changes account for this slower growth, according to Joseph Hafkenschiel, executive director of the California Association for Health Services at Home. First was Medicare's reimbursement squeeze.

Unlike California's nursing home industry, which is dependent on Medi-Cal reimbursement, the state's HHAs receive little reimbursement from this source. Indeed, Medi-Cal dramatically underutilizes home health services, which account for only 0.1 percent of the state's Medi-Cal budget. Because HHAs are so dependent on Medicare reimbursement, said Hafkenschiel, HCFA reimbursement policies have hurt the industry. Early in the 1980s, HCFA began to decrease the amount it would pay for home health visits; and, more important, beginning in 1986, the agency's fiscal intermediaries significantly increased the number of claim denials. In 1983, California HHAs provided an average of 17.3 visits per patient; by 1987, this number had dropped to 12.5 per patient.

Improved technology and the sophistication of home care have also led to some consolidation. Given the need for specialized equipment and personnel, HHAs today are administratively more complex and require greater capital investment, than in the past, making it difficult for small HHAs to operate. Many of these HHAs did not have sufficient "capital, referral base, or expertise," Hafkenschiel believes.

Finally, competition and the new reimbursement system have made it difficult for some HHAs to survive. Sharon Grisby, president of the Visiting Nurses Association of Los Angeles (VNA-LA), stated in a January 1989 interview that HHAs compete for hospital contracts. Further, like hospitals, they contract with HMOs and PPOs, all of which want "discounts," Grisby said.

Competition is also fierce for nurses. Because the VNA-LA pays 5 percent to 8 percent less than hospitals, it had a 40 percent turnover in nurses during 1988.

Access and Quality. Medi-Cal patients find it even more difficult obtaining home health care than finding nursing home placements. Medi-Cal not only significantly underpays for home health visits; it also sets up a number of administrative hurdles before authorization for home health services can be obtained.

The VNA-LA is one of only about ten California agencies accepting Medi-Cal patients, according to Sharon Grisby. Other Los Angeles HHAs limit their Medi-Cal patient load to 2 percent or take a case or two as a favor to a provider, but generally the VNA gets all the Medi-Cal referrals.

"The VNA has a monopoly on Medi-Cal," Grisby complained. Medi-Cal patients are unattractive to home health agencies for three reasons. First, the program does not pay enough to cover the costs of patient visits. It costs the VNA-LA $75 for an average visit, but Medi-Cal pays only $62. By contrast, Medicare pays up to $75–$78 a visit. Second, Medi-Cal has a disproportionate number of "high tech" cases, including AIDS patients: In 1988, 20 percent of the VNA-LA patient load was Medi-Cal, but 40 percent of the agency's high-tech visits were for Medi-Cal patients. A specialized visit, which requires more time and the resources of more highly trained nurses, costs an average of $99. And third, Medi-Cal, like Medicare, will often arbitrarily deny claims.

Both hospital administrators and HHA representatives interviewed for this study agreed that over the 1980s the acuity of home care increased dramatically. The PPS had a profound effect on home health care. "High-tech care has moved from hospital to home," declared Grisby. She continued by saying that, today, "even the routine med-surg cases are train wrecks. Ten years ago the bread-and-butter cases were new diabetes, stabilized stroke patients, post surgical patients who were all but healed. [Now,] we don't even see [what had been a] mainstay case ten years ago." Instead, the VNA-LA sees "brittle diabetes [diabetes that has not been stabilized]. New diabetics are sent home from the hospital with a brochure."

This higher acuity increases the costs of care. The VNA-LA, for example, no longer hires new nursing graduates because they do not have the skills and experience that specialty care requires.

However, it is the overwhelming consensus of persons interviewed for this study that higher acuity of home care patients has not resulted from inappropriate discharges. Grisby said that it "doesn't happen very frequently" that a patient is discharged inappropriately. "If a patient is too sick for the VNA," there is usually no problem with "utilization review." Hafkenschiel of the California Association of Health Services at Home concurred with this assessment. "I'm not hearing that home health patients are not so sick that they shouldn't be home."

Hospice Care

In the health care industry, services follow reimbursement. Medicare's 1983 decision to add hospice care as a reimbursable service and the decision of private insurers to follow suit led to a significant expansion of hospice services in Los Angeles, especially by hospital home care agencies. Medi-Cal began reimbursing for hospice care in 1988.

Hospice care is provided by a number of different organizations. Because hospice agencies are not licensed per se, any organization or entrepreneur can call itself a hospice. However, for Medicare and Medi-Cal reimbursement, hospice certification is required. For the most part, hospice care is provided under the auspices of hospital-based and independent home health agencies.

Generally, the hospice services available in Los Angeles meet only part of the county's needs. Only three hospices (one of them a Kaiser facility available only to its members) with a total of eighty-five beds are licensed to provide both residential and medical care. A new category of licensure established by the state in 1988, congregate-living health facilities for the terminally ill, may encourage the growth of more residential services for the terminally ill with no homes.

Physicians

The 1980s were a time of change and some consternation for Los Angeles physicians. They saw the traditional fee-for-service practice give way under the onslaught of the new HMO/PPO competitive environment. In addition, they saw greater scrutiny by insurers, pressure by hospital administrators to change hospital practices, and a different entrepreneurial ethic that encouraged investment in a host of for-profit health care enterprises.

Physician Growth/Maldistribution. Los Angeles has enough physicians to care for its population. In 1985, Los Angeles County had 227 physicians for every 100,000 people. Between 1980 and 1985, the number of physicians in the county increased by 17 percent.

However, Los Angeles physicians are seriously maldistributed by both specialty and geography. Despite the need for more primary care physicians, the percent of Los Angeles physicians in general practice specialties increased only slightly from 1980 to 1985, from 10.1 to 10.3 percent, and it does not seem likely that the percent of primary care physicians will increase in the near future. Robert Tranquada, dean of the USC School of Medicine, has the impression that the number of residency applications in areas such as pediatrics and internal medicine has declined recently. Although this decline may not make sense in terms of societal need, it makes "economic sense," he said, because the "noncognitive areas" of medicine are still doing well financially.

In Los Angeles, as in all large urban U.S. communities, in the midst of plenty, there is scarcity. White middle- and upper-class communities have more physicians than needed, whereas poor black and Latino communities are starved for physicians. The disparity between physician-rich and physician-poor communities in Los Angeles is great.

Table 4.3 presents physician distribution data for selected Los Angeles communities. As the table shows, communities with large, white upper-income populations, such as Beverly Hills, West Los Angeles, Santa Monica, and Sherman Oaks, have far more physicians than are needed. Yet the residents of largely poor minority communities, such as El Monte, East

TABLE 4.3   Population/Physician Ratios and Physician Characteristics in Selected Communities in Los Angeles County, 1984–1986

	Beverly Hills	El Monte	East L.A.	West L.A.	Santa Monica	Sherman Oaks	Watts
Population/ physician	125	2,216	873	1,189	220	359	613
Population/ primary care physician	344	2,918	1,300	396	589	867	1,244
Population/ obstetrician	2,341	23,928	57,204	3,803	3,969	8,674	6,530
Population/ pediatrician	2,838	13,293	9,534	1,849	4,481	4,994	4,353
Population/ surgeon	559	19,940	9,534	683	1,120	2,022	4,664
Percent of Black physicians	2	4	2	1	−1	1	41
Percent of Latino physicians	1	12	23	1	1	2	5
Percent of FMG physicians	18	57	46	17	13	24	33

Source: California Office of Statewide Health Planning and Development, Characteristics of Physicians Licensed by the California Board of Medical Quality Assurance, July 1984 through June 1986, July 1988.

Los Angeles, and Watts, have few physicians to care for them. For example, Beverly Hills has one practicing physician for every 125 residents; El Monte has one physician for every 2,216 residents. The physician disparity between rich and poor, white and minority communities applies to primary-care physicians and to all specialities. El Monte, with a population of 119,639, has only six surgeons located within its borders.

These communities also differ in the percentages of practicing minority physicians and physicians who graduated from foreign medical schools. In the largely Latino communities of El Monte and East Los Angeles, 12 percent and 23 percent, respectively, of the practicing physicians are Latino, and 57 percent and 46 percent, respectively, are graduates of foreign medical schools; in Beverly Hills and West Los Angeles, only 1 percent of the physicians are Latino and fewer than 18 percent are graduates of foreign medical schools (Table 4.3).

Nurses

As discussed in earlier sections of this chapter, hospitals, insurers, HMOs, nursing homes, and nursing registries in Los Angeles fiercely compete for nurses. Efforts are being made on a number of fronts to increase the supply of nurses. UCLA, for example, is rapidly expanding the number of nursing students it can train and has instituted an outreach program to high school and junior college students.

Southern California hospitals joined together under the auspices of the Hospital Council of Southern California to form a Health Careers Information Center, which opened in November 1988. The hospitals hope that through its media campaign and clearinghouse, the center can recruit high school students and adults seeking new careers to enter nursing and other programs in the health professions.

As previously discussed, the lack of nurses is a particular problem for the Los Angeles Department of Health Services. Poor working conditions and low wages were the major causes of a nursing strike in February 1988 at the largest county hospital, LAC/USC Medical Center. The strike closed the hospital to everything but emergency room care. Nurses have since been given unprecedented attention in the form of pay raises, and some hospitals have even taken steps to improve working conditions, a long-standing demand of nursing leaders and the rank and file.

Public Policy

The Problems Drive the Politics

Throughout the 1980s, California was battered by the growing number of people who were completely uninsured for health care expenses, by the shrinking public capacity to provide health care to its low income uninsured and Medicaid population, and by the soaring costs for health care and for health insurance.

Today, a widespread and growing perception that the problem of the uninsured has reached crisis proportions has brought health care reform to the forefront of the political agenda. Leaders of business, labor, the hospital industry, the medical profession, the health insurance industry, the legislature, and the state government, as well as advocates for the low-income uninsured population, agreed that the system is in serious trouble. Many of the most active leaders believe that California's health care financing system is on a slippery slope headed toward collapse. Each constituency leader sees the problem from his or her own perspective, defining the probable catastrophe differently and identifying somewhat different causes and remedies, but all are convinced that the growing uninsured population and the ever escalating health care costs are the core of the problem. And each believes public policy action is urgently needed. However, no political consensus has emerged concerning the reforms that should be enacted.

What the State Has Done

California has expanded its already generous Medi-Cal eligibility and could expand it slightly more. But with one of the most generous Medicaid eligibility standards in the country, there is not a lot of room left to cover the uninsured using this joint state-federal program. Furthermore, the fact that any individual is eligible for Medi-Cal does not guarantee access because the program pays providers so little and burdens them with so many restrictions that most doctors refuse to treat more than a few Medi-Cal patients. Expanding eligibility and raising payments to providers would dramatically increase the costs of the Medi-Cal program.

The risk pool enacted in California in 1991 may provide some relief for people who have been denied health insurance because of preexisting medical conditions, but only if they are very affluent. The three PPO health plans offered through the program provide modest benefits, require substantial deductibles and copayments, and cap the plan's benefits at $50,000 a year, a not overly generous provision for beneficiaries who may be at risk for catastrophic medical expenses. For the program to provide even this level of coverage, the state is subsidizing it with tobacco tax dollars, which has enabled premiums to be reduced to 125 percent of standard-risk individual policies. Although this approach has a lot of appeal because it targets people whose desperate need for coverage is obvious even to the most skeptical observer, the plan's high costs are expected to keep out all but 15,000 of the estimated 244,000 medically uninsurable persons in California.

California also enacted in 1991 and plans to implement in 1993 a modest program of tax credits to encourage small employers to offer health insurance coverage to their employees. The participation by small employers is likely to be influenced by the very factors that discourage them from providing this fringe benefit: low profit margins and the cost of the insurance. These factors add up to a competitive disadvantage for those who would increase their labor costs for the products or services they must sell. Few small employers are likely to buy into such a program because the cost of benefits remains high and participation remains voluntary. In the end, relatively few of the uninsured can be expected to participate in and benefit from the recently enacted program.

Remaining Public Policy Options

The approaches to the problem of the uninsured being considered range from proposals that would extend access to insurance coverage to some groups of the uninsured—an incremental, targeted strategy—to proposals that would provide insurance to the entire population and substantially or completely reform the financing of health care in the state by establishing a universal health services financing program. The incremental approach includes the modest programs and policies already enacted in California, as well as some additional proposals. The most dramatic incremental policy option under consideration would require employers to provide health benefits to their employees or, a "play or pay" alternative, to require employers who do not provide health benefits to pay a tax to a state-sponsored coverage program. The employer-mandate proposals have received some political support from medical industry groups, including the politically powerful California Medical Association, but business groups have vehemently attacked them and consumer groups have been less than enthusiastic.

Health Access, a statewide consumer coalition, has proposed a total reform of the health care financing system in California. Its proposal recommends the financing of a comprehensive package of health services through a largely tax-funded system rather than through insurance premiums and large out-of-pocket payments, as most health care services are financed today. The proposal would end the dependence of health insurance coverage on employment. The entire population would be covered in one program, and each person would be able to enroll in a variety of prepaid health plans or opt to go the doctor of his or her choice under a state-run health insurance program. This proposal, although taken seriously by major political forces in the state, has a narrow base of active support. Health Access has not convinced business or most labor unions to climb on its bandwagon.

The 1992 election in California may be an important milestone if, as many expect, Health Access and the California Medical Association take their competing proposals to the ballot through the initiative process. Recent national public opinion polls have found support for national health insurance among about two thirds of adult respondents, and support is even stronger in California, where the uninsured problem is more severe. In a poll in Orange County, an area of California that is not noted for its liberal politics, 75 percent of the respondents favored national health insurance, including 67 percent of the Republicans surveyed. Nevertheless, the failure of most initiatives on the 1990 election ballot has raised concern among reform advocates that this path may not be a viable road to success. Modified proposals are being considered by a number of groups involved in these public policy deliberations, including Health Access and the California Medical Association.

Summing Up

The political dilemma in California is apparent. Like the country as a whole, the state has two problems that are inextricably linked: a large uninsured population and rapidly rising health care costs. Political support is growing rapidly to enact public policies that would extend access to health care to the uninsured and underinsured population. At the same time, there is great concern that new coverage would add a costly program to the state's already desperate fiscal problems or add costs to private businesses and fuel inflation in health care prices and total expenditures. The federal government and Congress have essentially abrogated any significant role in solving these problems; in the absence of national leadership, California, like other states, feels it is on its own.

Major health care financing reforms are possible in California through either the legislative or the initiative process. Because of the give-and-take in the legislative process and because this process allows problems in programmatic and policy proposals to be somewhat more easily corrected, a legislative solution to the state's health care crisis is clearly preferable. But California, like most states and the national political structure, is burdened with a legislative process that is more suited to interest-group intervention and control than it is to solving social problems. Unhindered by the morass that has impeded the legislative process in California, the initiative process seems a more attractive and more likely way to solve the state's health care problems. This form of direct democracy, available in some states but not at the national level, may be the most viable avenue by which to avoid the legislative gridlock that blocks significant health care reform.

Nevertheless, as Los Angeles and California enter the 1990s, the chances for health care reform in the short term are not encouraging. In the meantime, the poor and middle-income populations will see their access to affordable health care eroded further. Hospitals and physicians will face increased pressure to reduce costs. During the 1980s, the health care system in Los Angeles County underwent a dramatic transformation, one that benefitted neither providers nor consumers. Only if greater political power and leadership are mobilized on behalf of significant health care reform will the increasing turmoil and crisis of the past decade be avoided in the 1990s.

Bibliography

Andresky, J., "The Mess at Maxicare," Forbes, June 27, 1988.
Applegate, J., "Owners Must Face New Workplace Concerns, " Los Angeles Times, January 13, 1989, Part IV, 3.
Blendon, R.J., Taylor, H., "Views on Health Care: Public Opinion in Three Nations," Health Affairs 8 (Spring 1989): 149–157.
Blue Cross of California, About Blue Cross of California (Los Angeles: Blue Cross, 1987).

Boyarsky, B., "Budget Calls for Medical Aid Cuts for L.A. County's Poor," *Los Angeles Times*, January 11, 1989, Part I, 15.

Braun, S., "County Mental Centers Reject 50% of Cases, Study Finds," *Los Angeles Times*, June 1, 1988, Part II, 3.

Brown, E.R., *Public Medicine in Crisis: Public Hospitals in California*, California Policy Seminar Monograph No. 11 (Berkeley: Institute for Governmental Studies, University of California, 1981).

Brown, E.R., Cousineau, M.R., Price, W.T., "Competing for Medi-Cal Business: Why Hospitals Did, and Did Not, Get Contracts." *Inquiry* 22 (1985): 237–250.

Brown, E.R., Price, W.T., Cousineau, M.R., "Medi-Cal Hospital Contracting: Did It Achieve Its Legislative Objectives? " *Western Journal of Medicine* 143 (1985): 118–124.

Brown, E.R., Valdez, R.B., Morgenstern, H., Bradley, T., Hafner, C., *Californians Without Health Insurance: A Report to the California Legislature* (Berkeley: California Policy Seminar, University of California, 1987).

Brown, E.R., Valdez, R.B., Morgenstern, H., Cumberland, W., Wang, C., Mann, J., *Health Insurance Coverage of Californians in 1989* (Berkeley: California Policy Seminar, University of California, 1991).

Brown, E.R., Valdez, R.B., Morgenstern, H., Nourjah, P., Hafner, C., *Changes in Health Insurance Coverage of Californians, 1979–1986* (Berkeley: California Policy Seminar, University of California, 1988).

Bry, B., "Hospital Management Firms in Good Health and May Get Even Better," *Los Angeles Times*, May 3, 1981, Part IV, 1, 11, 13.

California Association of Hospitals and Health Systems (CAHHS), *1988 Hospital Fact Book* (Sacramento: CAHHS, 1988).

California Department of Health Services, *Health Data Summaries for California Counties, 1980*, and *Health Data Summaries for California Counties, 1988* (Sacramento: California Department of Health Services, 1980, 1988).

———. Center of Health Statistics, *Health Data Summaries for California Counties, 1980* (Sacramento: California Department of Health Services, 1980).

California Licensing and Certification Division, State Department of Health Services, *Statement of Deficiencies and Plan of Correction*, Los Angeles County/USC Medical Center, July 10, 1989.

———. State Department of Health Services, *Statement of Deficiencies and Plan of Correction*, Martin Luther King Medical Center, June 28, 1989.

California Major Risk Medical Insurance Program, *1991 Health Plans* (Sacramento: California Major Risk Medical Insurance Program, 1991).

California Medical Assistance Commission, *Listing of Hospitals That Have Had Contracts with Effective Date of Contracting and/or Termination as of December 1, 1989*—For Los Angeles County (Sacramento: California Medical Assistance Commission, 1989).

California Office of Statewide Health Planning and Development (OSHPD), *Individual Long-Term Care Facility Financial Data, Report Periods Ending December 31, 1987–December 30, 1988*, Vol. 2 (Sacramento: OSHPD, 1989).

———. *Quarterly Individual Hospital Data for California, 3rd Quarter, 1988*, Vol. 2 (Sacramento: OSHPD, 1988).

_____ . *Licensed Services and Utilization Profiles: Annual Report of Hospitals* (Sacramento: OSHPD, 1987-1988).

_____ . "Trends in Home Health Agency Openings and Closings" (Sacramento: OSHPD, 1986).

_____ . *Annual Report of Home Health Agencies* (Sacramento: OSHPD, 1985, 1986, 1987, 1988).

_____ . *Characteristics of Physicians Licensed by the California Board of Medical Quality Assurance* (Sacramento: OSHPD, 1984, 1985, 1986, 1988) .

Communicable Disease Morbidity Report, County of Los Angeles, 1987 (Los Angeles: Department of Health Services, 1987).

Community and Organizational Research Institute, University of California, Santa Barbara, *1982–1986 Maternal and Child Health Data Base* (Santa Barbara: UCSB, 1989).

County Fact Book, '88-'89 (Sacramento: County Supervisors Association of California, 1989).

Cousineau, M.R., Brown, E.R., Freedman, J.E., "Access to Free Care for Indigent Patients in Los Angeles: County Policy Implementation and Barriers to Care." *Journal of Ambulatory Care Management* 10 (1987): 78–89.

Dallek, G., *The Quality of Medical Care for the Poor in Los Angeles County's Health and Hospital System* (Los Angeles: Legal Aid Foundation of Los Angeles, 1987).

Davidson, S.M., "Physician Participation in Medicaid: Background and Issues." *Journal of Health Politics, Policy and Law* 6 (1982): 703–717.

"For Some HMOs, the Risk of Medicare Is Paying Off," *Modern Healthcare*, January 13, 1989, 47–48.

Garcia, K.J., "Panel Delays Vote on King Hospital Accreditation," *Los Angeles Times*, January 13, 1990, part B, 3, 8.

_____ . "Obstetric Care Crisis at Hand for County," *Los Angeles Times*, December 29, 1989, part B, 1, 8.

_____ . "Turnaround by King Hospital Rescues Funds," *Los Angeles Times*, December 19, 1989, A1, 17.

Garner, D.D., Liao, W.C., Sharpe, T.R., "Factors Affecting Physician Participation in a State Medicaid Program," *Medical Care* 17 (1979): 43–58.

Gates, R., *AIDS—Report for June 1989* (Los Angeles: Department of Health Services, 1989).

_____ . *Fiscal Year 1988-89 and 1989-90 Budget Policy Issues—Department of Health Services* (Los Angeles: Department of Health Services, 1988, 1989).

Gordon, L., "'Bed Pan Alley': Health Care Facilities Changing Character of Hollywood's East Side," *Los Angeles Times*, August 15, 1985, Part II, 1, 6.

Grant, P., "Emergence of the California Health System," *California Hospitals*, January/February 1990, 48–49.

_____ . "What the History of California's Health System Tells Us About Its Future," *California Hospitals*, November/December 1989, 6–10.

Hadley, J., "Physician Participation in Medicaid: Evidence from California," *Health Services Research* 14 (1979): 266–280.

Hospital Council of Southern California, *Compensation Survey Report: Registered Nurses, 1989* (Los Angeles: Hospital Council of Southern California, 1989).

_____ . *Trend in Hospital Financial Results, Occupancy and Discharges: Hospitals in Los Angeles County First Quarter Results 1985 to 1988* (Los Angeles: Hospital Council of Southern California, 1985–1988).

"Insider Interview: Dr. Robert Gumbiner, Chairman and CEO, FHP Inc.," *HealthWeek*, October 31, 1988, 25.

Johns, L., "Selective Contracting in California: An Update," *Inquiry* 26 (Fall 1989): 345–353.

_____ . "Implications for Selective Contracting," *California Health Association Insight* 9 (September 16, 1985): 1–6.

Johnson, "Nursing Registries Booming; Some Say Trend Is Unhealthy," *Los Angeles Times*, June 4, 1989, Part II, 1, 2.

Kim, H., "Turnaround Specialist: California CEO Knows How to Heal Ailing Hospitals," *Modern Healthcare*, December 15, 1989, 56.

Knowles, R., "Doctors Criticized for Report," *Los Angeles Outlook*, August 19, 1987, A3.

Koetting, M., Olinger, L., "Selective Contracting in California: The First Year," *Medicaid Program Evaluation: Final Report*, chap. V (Washington, D.C.: Health Care Financing Administration, 1987).

Lazarus, W., Tirengel, J., *Back to Basics 1988: Strategies for Investing in the Health of California's Next Generation* (Los Angeles: Southern California Child Health Network, 1988).

Lazarus, W., West, K.M., *Back to Basics: Improving the Health of California's Next Generation* (Los Angeles: Southern California Child Health Network, 1987).

Levit, K.R., "Personal Health Care Expenditures, by State: 1966–82," *Health Care Financing Review* 6 (Summer 1985): 1–49.

Lewin, L., Ekels, T., Miller, L., "Setting the Record Straight: The Provision of Uncompensated Care by Not-for-Profit Hospitals," *New England Journal of Medicine* 318 (1988): 1212–1215.

Los Angeles County Department of Health Services, *How to Get No-Cost or Low-Cost Medical Care at County Hospitals and Clinics* (Los Angeles: Department of Health Services, 1989).

_____ . Data Collection and Analysis Division, *STD Clinic Attendance and Patient Attitude Survey* (Los Angeles: Department of Health Services, 1989).

_____ . *Draft Strategic Plan: 1988–1992* (Los Angeles: Department of Health Services, 1987).

_____ . *Evaluating the Effect of Charging for Prenatal Care in a Local Health Department*, Mimeograph (Los Angeles: Department of Health Services, 1987).

Los Angeles Homeless Health Care Project, *A Directory of Free and Community Clinics in Los Angeles* (Los Angeles: Homeless Health Care Project, 1989).

Lu, E., "Closure to Leave 1 Trauma Unit for San Gabriel Valley," *Los Angeles Times*, November 1, 1988, Part II, 1, 3.

Lurie, N., Ward, N.B., Shapiro, M.F., Brook, R.H., "Termination from Medi-Cal: Does It Affect Health?" *New England Journal of Medicine* 311 (1984): 480–484.

Lurie, N., Ward, N.B., Shapiro, M.F., Gallego, C., Vaghaiwalla, R., Brook, R.H., "Termination of Medi-Cal Benefits: A Follow-Up Study One Year Later," *New England Journal of Medicine* 314 (1986): 1266–1268.

Lutz, S., "Ambulatory Care Keeps Patients, Hospitals on the Move," *Modern Healthcare*, December 1, 1989, 32.

Mazely, S., *Perinatal Research Project: A Profile of the Obstetrical Patient Los Angeles County Health Care System* (Los Angeles: Department of Health Services, 1987).

Melnick, G.A., Mann, J., and Golan, I., "Uncompensated Emergency Care in Hospital Markets in Los Angeles County," *American Journal of Public Health* 79 (April 1989): 514–516.

Melnick, G.A., Zwanziger, J., "Hospital Behavior Under Competition and Cost-Containment Policies: The California Experience, 1980–1985," *Journal of the American Medical Association* 260 (1988): 2669–2675.

O'Shaugnessy, L., "Mental Health Clinic Closures Create Turmoil," *Los Angeles Times*, June 10, 1989, Part I, 1, 31.

Ong, P.M., et al. (eds.), *The Widening Divide: Income Inequality and Poverty in Los Angeles* (Los Angeles: Research Group on the Los Angeles Economy, UCLA Graduate School of Architecture and Urban Planning, 1989).

Oppenheim, et al., *Problems with Placement of Medi-Cal Patients in Nursing Homes in the Santa Monica Area* (Santa Monica: Santa Monica Area Health Action Coalition and the Commission on Older Americans of the City of Santa Monica, 1987).

Parachini, A., "Health Care Debate: Who Will Pay the Way?" *Los Angeles Times*, August 30, 1987.

Pattison, R.V., Katz, H.M., "Investor-Owned and Not-for-Profit Hospitals: A Comparison Based on California Data," *New England Journal of Medicine* 309 (1983): 347–353.

Peterson, S., "Poll: 75% in OC Favor National Health Insurance," *Orange County Register*, September 22, 1987, A1, A10–11.

Phillips, D., *A Health Insurance Pool for High Risk Californians–AB 600* (Sacramento: Assembly Office of Research, 1988).

Pokorny, G., "Report Card on Health Care," *Health Management Quarterly* 10 (1988): 3–7.

Reich, K., "Allstate's Dropping of Small Group Health Coverage Stings Many," *Los Angeles Times*, July 15, 1989, Part II, 1, 4.

Reich, K., "No Choice but to Cut Benefits, Hike Premiums, Blue Cross Says," *Los Angeles Times*, August 9, 1988, Part I, 3, 17.

Robinson, J.C., Luft H.S., "Competition, Regulation, and Hospital Costs, 1982–1986," *Journal of the American Medical Association* 260 (1988): 2676–2681.

Rosenblatt, R., Spiegel, C., "Half of State's Nursing Homes Fall Short in Federal Study," *Los Angeles Times*, December 2, 1988, Part I, 3, 34.

Rosner, D., *A Once Charitable Enterprise: Hospitals and Health Care in Brooklyn and New York, 1885–1915* (Cambridge: Cambridge University Press, 1982).

Scott, J., "Rise in Infant Deaths Laid to Drugs, Prenatal Neglect," *Los Angeles Times*, February 3, 1990, part A, 1, 33.

———. "Syphilis Cases in Infants May Be Underreported," *Los Angeles Times*, December 1, 1988, Part II, 1, 4.

"Selected Characteristics of HMOs by State and Plan Name," *The InterStudy Edge* 4 (1989): 29–30.

Shiver, J., "State Bars Watts Health Unit from Seeking Members," *Los Angeles Times,* March 25, 1987, Part II, 1, 6.

——— . "Health-Care Costs Rising Faster, Study Shows," *Los Angeles Times,* August 27, 1986, Part IV, 1, 4.

——— . "Health Firms Go Under the Budget Knife," *Los Angeles Times,* July 20, 1986, Part IV, 1, 5.

Simon, R., "Some Money Restored, But 2 Mental Clinics Will Close," *Los Angeles Times,* September 27, 1989, Part II, 1.

——— . "County Seeks to Cope with Governor's Cut in Funds," *Los Angeles Times,* July 8, 1989, Part II, 1, 10.

Sofaer, S., Rundall, T.G., Zeller, W.L., "Restrictive Reimbursement Policies and Uncompensated Care in California Hospitals, 1981–1986" (paper delivered at the American Public Health Association annual meeting, Boston, November 1988).

Southwick, K., "Blue Cross of California Slices Deficits as Big Losses Continue," *HealthWeek,* October 26, 1987, 4, 37.

Spiegel, C., "Demand for Prenatal Care Bogs Down Public Clinics," *Los Angeles Times,* November 8, 1989, Part I, 1.

——— . "Private Practice Strains Public Medicine at King," *Los Angeles Times,* September 4, 1989, Part I, 1, 30–31.

——— . "Hospital: A Crisis in Critical Care," *Los Angeles Times,* September 3, 1989, Part I, 1, 34–36.

——— . "Debate Continues on Future of Besieged Trauma Center," *Los Angeles Times,* August 22, 1989, Part II, 1, 8.

——— . "Options Fading Fast for L.A. County Burn Victims," *Los Angeles Times,* August 4, 1989, Part I, 1, 3, 39.

——— . "Doctors' Use of Own Labs: Good Ethics?" *Los Angeles Times,* February 17, 1989, Part I, 1, 22.

——— . "'Medical Gridlock' Hits County's Emergency Rooms," *Los Angeles Times,* January 18, 1989, Part II, 1, 8.

——— . "X-Ray Workers Join Nurse Strikes; Doctors May Walk," *Los Angeles Times,* January 29, 1988, Part I, 1, 4.

Spiegel, C., Hurst, J., "Nursing Homes: Medi-Cal Rules Abet Poor Care," *Los Angeles Times,* April 8, 1988, Part A, 1, 27, 31.

Spiegel, C., Scott, J., "Hospital Merger Will Close Aging Queen of Angels," *Los Angeles Times,* November 4, 1988, Part I, 1, 26.

Spiegel, C., Steinbrook, R., "Emergency Room Cutbacks Set Off Debate on Causes," *Los Angeles Times,* May 8, 1989, Part I, 1, 5.

Starr, L.M., Hospital Council of Southern California, *AIDS Survey Report* (Los Angeles: Hospital Council of Southern California, 1988).

Steinbrook, R., Spiegel, C., "California Private Hospitals Low in Charity Services," *Los Angeles Times,* May 5, 1988, Part II, 1, 6.

Steinbrook, R., Vickers, R.J., "Medicare Mortality Rates: 72 Facilities Top Predictions," *Los Angeles Times,* December 21, 1989, part A, 3, 42.

Taravella, S., "Market Focus: Los Angeles," *Modern Healthcare* (September 8, 1989): 32–37.

——— . "Success in Treating the Poor," *Modern Healthcare* (September 8, 1989): 48.

Vollmer, T., "County Acts to Cut Alien Medical Tab: Illegals Will Have to Apply for Medi-Cal to Receive Treatment," *Los Angeles Times*, April 16, 1986, Part II, 1.

Warren, J., "Resurgence of Measles Kills 6 in California," *Los Angeles Times*, February 2, 1990, part A, 1, 24.

White, G., "The Uninsured: Health Gamble Affects 1 in 5," *Los Angeles Times*, January 29, 1990, part A, 1, 16.

Williams, L., "AMI to Move Its Headquarters from Beverly Hills to Dallas," *Los Angeles Times*, December 22, 1989, part D, 1, 6.

———. "Maxicare Loses $169.7 Million in Quarter, Blames Costly Writeoffs," *Los Angeles Times*, December 7, 1988, Part IV, 1, 15.

Woutat, D., "Maxicare's Ills Fuel Debate Over Benefits of HMOs," *Los Angeles Times*, March 20, 1989, Part IV, 1, 9.

Zonana, V.F., "AIDS Fight in L.A. at Key Point," *Los Angeles Times*, December 31, 1989, part A, 1, 36, 37.

5

The Shifting Mosaic of Health and Medical Care in Houston and Harris County, Texas, in the Late 1980s

Hardy D. Loe, Jr., Virginia C. Kennedy, and Frank I. Moore

The compelling story in health and health care in the United States in the last quarter-century has been the conflict between controlling the rising cost of care and assuring access to services, quality of care, and health status gains. In the immediate post–World War II era the nation was prosperous, confronted with institutions severely neglected by the Great Depression and the war and poised for the expansion of health systems and services. For two decades, improving access to health care was pursued without concern for the availability of resources. Facilities were increased with the federal Hill-Burton program, private health insurance mushroomed as benefits were included in collective bargaining packages, federal grants-in-aid to public health departments increased, health manpower training was subsidized and significant participation by the federal government in the financing of biomedical research began. At the end of the second decade, the passage of Medicare and Medicaid signaled the last major initiative in the quest for access to health care, and within a few years, the nation began to realize that resources were limited and cost controls were necessary. The evolving planning, regulatory, and reimbursement policies and procedures that continue to this day have stimulated profound changes, although the goal of a health care system that offers quality care to all citizens in need at reasonable cost remains elusive.

This chapter provides a window through which we can view how attempts to resolve these issues are being played out in Houston and Harris County, Texas. The observations are quite recent and reflect the dynamic and rapidly changing nature of these relationships. A major theme in the Harris County experience is the reluctance within the health sector to grant a major role to government at any level in its operations and the corresponding preference for entrepreneurship at both the practitioner and institutional level.

Background

Population and Economy

Houston, with a 1990 population of 1.6 million, is the largest city in Texas and the fourth largest city in the United States. It is the county seat of Harris County, whose 1990 population totaled 2.8 million, and is the center of the ninth largest Consolidated Metropolitan Statistical Area (CMSA) in the nation, a seven-county region containing 3.8 million persons. The land area encompassed by these entities, and the associated geographic distances, are large. The CMSA, for example, is nearly equal in square mileage to the state of New Jersey, and the city of Houston alone is more than one-half the size of Rhode Island. The health care needs and the geographical dispersion of this large population are important determinants of the characteristics and distribution of the health care system that serves it.

The Houston CMSA experienced a population increase of nearly 20 percent between 1980 and 1990. The highest rate of growth, however, occurred outside of Houston; the city's population increased by only about 2 percent. The average age of Houston's residents increased slightly during the 1980s, but with the median age estimated at 30.3 years in 1989, the region's population was relatively young in comparison to other large CMSAs. Although the health problems of the young predominate, there is a large population of elders whose illness experiences also influence health service delivery requirements.

The 1980s produced major changes in the racial and ethnic composition of Houston and the surrounding region. The number of Anglos, or non-Hispanic whites, residing in Houston decreased by more than one-fifth, while the number residing in the CMSA outside the city of Houston increased by nearly one-fourth. By 1990, Anglos constituted 40 percent of Houston's population, down from 53 percent in 1980. The economic losses to the tax base that other communities experienced with the out-migration of Anglo populations were blunted in Houston because of a state law that allows the easy annexation by cities of adjacent communities. The number of Hispanics in Houston increased from 18 to 28 percent of the population during this period; the proportion of blacks remained unchanged at 28 percent. The Asian population doubled, constituting 4 percent of the city's residents in 1990. Because Houston's population comprises large numbers of minorities, the cultural determinants of access to, and effectiveness of, health services are important considerations.

Major industries in the Houston area include shipping, petrochemical and other manufacturing, agriculture, medical care, and other service industries. The National Aeronautics and Space Center at Clear Lake, twenty-five miles southeast of Houston, constitutes the area's major government industry. Although some fifty miles inland, Houston possesses the largest port in total annual tonnage shipped from the southern United States. The diversity of industry to some extent assures a strong economic base, but the propensity for accompanying environmental and occupational health hazards is present and evokes responses from both the private and the public health care sectors.

During the mid-1980s, the region experienced a major recession. Houston's gross area product, estimated in 1982 at $96.9 billion, dipped to $81.6 billion in 1987. Per capita personal income in the Houston CMSA, which was the eighth highest in the nation in 1983, ranked twenty-fifth in 1988. The unemployment rate in 1986, according to the Texas Employment Commission, was 10.3 percent. By 1988 the rate dropped to 6.8 percent and by May 1989 to 5.3 percent. The numbers of unemployed fell from 145,600 in 1986 to 97,900 in 1988. Recovery is attributed to the diversification of the economic base from one heavily dependent upon oil to one emphasizing the creation of small businesses, expanded international trade, and anticipated government contracts with the Space Center.

Economic recovery continues in the early 1990s. Although employment is up, a large number of the new jobs are in the service sector on a part-time and contractual basis. Many employed people do not receive fringe benefits, including health insurance. Several employers, especially the smaller ones, have discontinued health insurance as a fringe benefit altogether, so that the percentage of workers without health coverage is rising.

Minorities continue to face high levels of unemployment and lack opportunities to develop skills required for future jobs. Particularly hard hit are blacks, who in 1987 accounted for 15.2 percent of the civilian labor force but 36.8 percent of the unemployed, according to the U.S. Department of Labor.

Although economic projections reflect continuing improvement, newly created jobs will increasingly demand higher and more sophisticated skills. The poor and unskilled will face mounting difficulties in gaining or retaining the benefits of full-time jobs. The paradox of recovery is that economically vulnerable populations do not participate equitably in the improvement in the economy.

The Health Care Establishment

Houston/Harris County is a major health care area and referral point with a comprehensive inventory that includes more than 7,000 physicians, over 16,000 nurses, and a wide range of other health care personnel. Facilities encompass multispecialty and specialty group practices, sixty-four community hospitals, as well as long-term-care institutions and a large number of alternative care organizations. The public health care sector consists of a tax-supported county hospital district, which provides medical care to the indigent; the city health department; the county health department; the county mental health/mental retardation unit; and a county psychiatric hospital.

The hub of health care, teaching, and research is the Texas Medical Center (TMC), a massive complex of forty-one hospitals and academic institutions. Collectively, these institutions constitute a major source of employment in the area and exert a significant impact on the local economy.

Each institution in the TMC is independently managed. In the aggregate they are held in loose confederation by common real estate, parking, laundry, energy, and computer and other support services offered by TMC. The Medical Center provides a forum for voluntary interaction. Its purpose is to maintain an environment that encourages excellence in research and patient care. TMC institutions receive referrals from a large area of the United States as well as from international markets, especially those of Central and South America.

Two academic medical centers are located in the Texas Medical Center, Baylor College of Medicine and The University of Texas (UT) Health Science Center at Houston. Baylor College of Medicine encompasses, in addition to its medical school, a division of allied health professions, a graduate school, several large specialty research centers, and a unit to facilitate the dissemination of new technology. The University of Texas Health Science Center serves as an administrative umbrella for eight academic health science teaching and research institutions: the School of Allied Health Sciences, a dental branch, the Graduate School of Biomedical Sciences, a medical school, a school of nursing, a school of public health, a division of continuing education, and a speech and hearing institute. A significant, separate component of the UT system in the Texas Medical Center is The University of Texas System Cancer Center, which includes the M.D. Anderson Hospital and Tumor Institute.

Professional associations of practitioners in the Houston area include the Harris County Medical Society with approximately 6,200 active members (7,400, if students and retired physicians are counted); the Houston Medical Forum, a professional organization of black physicians (most of whom also belong to the Harris County Medical Society); the Houston

District Dental Society; the Charles George Dental Society (an organization of black dentists); and District 9 of the Texas Nurses Association. Numerous specialty societies and associations of other health professionals also exist.

An active hospital planning organization, the Greater Houston Hospital Council, has approximately eighty member hospitals, sixty-four of which are in Harris County and the remainder in fourteen surrounding counties. The council represents its members in a wide variety of legislative and public relations concerns, provides shared services such as group purchasing, coordinates hospital planning for the area, and maintains important statistical data bases.

Voluntary health agencies have long been an active and important part of the health establishment. Particularly prominent, among others, are the March of Dimes Birth Defects Foundation, the San Jacinto Lung Association, Planned Parenthood of America, the American Cancer Society, and the American Heart Association. As in other communities, their roles vary widely and include education, advocacy, the support of health services research, and the provision of health care.

The business community has organized the Houston Area Health Care Coalition, with a primary interest of which is finding ways to control medical care costs. The coalition collects data and, from time to time, publishes reports of interest to its members and the health care system at large. The coalition maintains an active interest in the public health sector as well.

Although organized labor is active in Harris County, the movement is not as strong as in other parts of the United States. Little formal union activity is directed toward health care issues.

In summary, Houston and Harris County have a pluralistic, loosely confederated health care establishment. Its capacity is large, its diversity is impressive, and it boasts high-quality service delivery. The health care system is an interesting mix of interdependence and independence. It makes significant contributions to meeting the health and medical care needs of the population of Harris County and beyond, extending to the region, the nation, and foreign countries.

The Private Sector

The majority of medical care encounters in Houston and Harris County occur in the private sector. Emergency care is an exception as it is provided primarily in emergency facilities of the public hospital system. The principal providers of care in the private sector are the hospitals, physicians, alternative delivery systems, and long-term-care facilities. Their characteristics, utilization, and interrelationships as well as the impact upon them of cost-containment pressures, reimbursement policies, and other stresses are important factors in understanding health and health care in Harris County.

The Acute-Care System

Hospital Ownership and Utilization. The principal dynamics of the hospital system in Houston/Harris County during the 1980s are reflected in statistical data maintained nationally by the American Hospital Association (AHA) and locally by the Greater Houston Hospital Council (GHHC). Some inconsistencies in data from the two sources are related to differences in the classification of facilities and the time of year that information was reported to each source, but trends in hospital capacity and utilization revealed by both sources are identical.

AHA data show an increase in the total number of hospitals in Houston and Harris County from fifty-four in 1976 to sixty-one in 1986. One year later the number decreased to fifty-nine. The corresponding number of beds for this period was 13,173 in 1976, increasing to a peak of 15,555 in 1982, and then declining to 15, 311 in 1986 and 15,090 in 1987. Although the number of hospitals reached a high point in 1986, the number of beds actually declined slightly in that year and has continued to decline modestly. These figures are low when compared to the figures in Table 5.1 from the Greater Houston Hospital Council. According to GHHC data, the total number of hospitals in the county was sixty-eight in 1987 and sixty-seven in 1989; the total number of beds was 18,142 and 18,094, respectively, for those years. The differences apparently are due to more complete reporting to the council than to the American Hospital Association.

In terms of ownership, Table 5.1 shows that the largest number of hospitals and the greatest number of beds are in for-profit systems and a few individually owned facilities. The ratio of for-profit beds to not-for-profit beds in 1987 was approximately 8.7 to 6. 3. This large number of for-profit facilities reflects a trend of hospital purchasing by for-profit systems that started in the late 1960s. By the early 1970s Houston was known as "acquisition city." Principal reasons given by industry representatives for this for-profit hospital growth are twofold: a competitive environment and unique investment opportunities.

Subsequently, this trend has lessened. AHA data show that the number of investor-owned hospitals increased from thirty-six to forty-two between 1976 and 1986 and the number of not-for-profit hospitals decreased from fourteen to thirteen. More recently, from 1987 to 1989, there was a net increase of only one investor-owned hospital and a decrease of two not-for-profit hospitals.

TABLE 5.1   Hospital Capacity and Ownership, Houston/Harris County, 1987 and 1989

	1987		1989	
	Hospitals	Beds	Hospitals	Beds
Investor-owned corporations	40	8,581	42	8,690
For-profit, single owner	4	310	3	293
Not-for-profit corporations	12	4,729	9	3,757
Not-for-profit independent	5	1,554	6	2,446
Government (public)	8	3,108	7	2,908
Total	68[a]	18,142[a]	67	18,094
Psychiatric	12	1,632	15	1,828

[a]One 140-bed public hospital is managed by a not-for-profit corporation. This hospital appears in both categories in the body of this table but is counted only once in the totals.

Source: Greater Houston Hospital Council.

Data on hospital beds by ownership show little change from 1987 to 1989. For-profit beds increased slightly from 8,891 to 8,983, and the number of not-for-profit hospital beds dropped slightly, from 6,283 to 6,203.

Occupancy rates in hospitals reporting to the AHA dropped dramatically between 1982 and 1986 from approximately 68 percent to about 50 percent. A slight increase in occupancy to around 52 percent occurred in 1987. Admissions declined steadily during this period from 369,500 in 1976 to 348,300 in 1982 to 332,100 in 1987. Similarly, length of stay declined from a peak of 7.4 days in 1982 to 6.9 in 1987.

These declines in utilization measures are attributed by most observers to the institution by Medicare of reimbursement based on diagnosis-related groups in 1983. Subsequently, other factors have played a role. Medicare and private insurance have become increasingly more restrictive in reimbursements for inpatient care. Insurers and the business coalition have exerted pressures on providers to shift services, both diagnostic and therapeutic, from the inpatient setting to less costly settings: outpatient, home-care, and long-term care facilities. For example, in response to fixed reimbursement per diagnosis-related group (DRG), health care facilities have decreased the number of days spent in the hospital per episode of illness (average length of stay) in favor of home care as a means of providing effective convalescence. Health maintenance organizations, as a matter of policy, limit both hospitalization and length of stay in favor of ambulatory care whenever possible.

With three notable exceptions, there was no new construction of acute care general hospitals during the late 1980s. The norm was to "downsize," that is, to close beds to admission as a means of paring both staffing and expenditures. Capacity was thus reduced consistent with the shortened average length of stay. The three exceptions were large teaching-research hospitals in the Texas Medical Center that are affiliated with the academic medical centers. All added beds and/or built additional facilities, such as professional buildings and ambulatory care centers. According to one informant, one of these hospitals attributes its continuing expansion and general profitability to the maintenance of a large international referral market.

Opinion is divided as to whether patient mix differs by payment source according to facility ownership. All levels of care and types of reimbursement are found in both for-profit and not-for-profit institutions, and some observers believe that there is no difference in patient mix in for-profit and not-for-profit hospitals. Others contend that Medicare and Medicaid are more readily accepted by not-for-profit facilities. The patient mix in the public hospital, which serves primarily indigent patients, is heavily skewed toward obstetrics and injuries as compared to the private hospitals' mix. The majority of patients are uninsured.

The Case of Psychiatric Hospitals. Psychiatric hospitals are also an exception to the "down-sizing" trend. Three new psychiatric hospitals opened between 1987 and 1989 (Table 5.1), accounting for an increase of 196 beds. Two of these were for-profit private hospitals and one was a county hospital operated in collaboration with The University of Texas Health Science Center. This expansion of psychiatric inpatient facilities and beds continues a trend that became evident in 1982, when six facilities were reported in Harris County, up from three in 1976. By 1987 there were nine.

The initial impetus for this expansion was the establishment of requirements by the State Insurance Board in 1981 for insurance carriers to increase coverage for alcohol and drug abuse problems. A second ruling in 1983 mandated broader psychiatric care coverage as well. This ruling stimulated private health insurance carriers to offer more liberal benefit packages for psychiatric illnesses. Other factors included the repeal of certificate-of-need legislation in 1983, the exemption of psychiatric conditions from diagnosis-related group reimbursement, a low requirement for capital investment, and the profitability of psychiatric care relative to general hospital care.

Insurance carriers have recently reduced benefits in the form of a thirty-day cap on inpatient coverage for any episode of psychiatric illness. In addition there is a growing trend by major corporations to reduce lifetime coverage for psychiatric care. Other pressures cited by a mental health administrator are the adverse decisions by utilization review organizations that may result in the reduction or denial of reimbursement.

These changes have been followed by a drop in occupancy rates in psychiatric facilities, and it remains to be seen whether the new units will remain financially viable under these conditions. The county psychiatric hospital, which has 250 beds and does not rely strictly on insurance revenues, has not followed the trend of reduced occupancy. Opened in 1989, the hospital quickly filled with patients and continues at capacity utilization.

The Academic Medical Centers. The two academic medical centers and their principal teaching hospitals are active participants in patient care, teaching, and research. Baylor College of Medicine, the older of the two, was established in Dallas in 1903 and was moved to Houston in 1943. The University of Texas Health Science Center at Houston (UTHSC-H) is relatively young; it opened its doors in 1972. Prior to that time, Baylor had teaching affiliations with four not-for-profit hospitals located in the Texas Medical Center and with the nearby Veterans Administration Hospital. Baylor also held a major contract to provide medical staff to the Harris County Hospital District, the public hospital and outpatient care institution in the county. With the opening of the UTHSC-H, those affiliations have changed somewhat. Baylor maintains its affiliations with three TMC acute-care facilities–Methodist Hospital, Texas Children's Hospital, and St. Luke's Episcopal Hospital–as well as with the Texas Institute for Rehabilitation and Research. The fourth major acute-care facility in the Texas Medical Center is Hermann Hospital, which is affiliated with UTHSC-H. UT also has affiliations with St. Joseph's Hospital in downtown Houston and with the Memorial Hospital System. The university's family practice residency program is housed at the Memorial Southwest Hospital facility located in southwest Houston. Both academic centers maintain limited affiliations with hospitals in other cities.

The two academic health centers also share arrangements with the public hospital system. Baylor retains its service and teaching affiliation with one of the system's major facilities, the Ben Taub Hospital, located in the TMC. The UTHSC-H has a similar service and teaching affiliation with the Harris County Hospital District's other newly constructed major facility, the Lyndon Baines Johnson Hospital, about twenty minutes away from the TMC in northeast Houston. The hospital district's network of neighborhood clinics is also shared between the two academic health centers.

The not-for-profit facilities associated with the academic medical centers fulfill multiple roles in the acute-care system in Harris County. First, like other acute-care general hospitals, these institutions provide primary hospital care for the patients of their respective medical staffs. In that sense they compete for patients with all other hospitals in Harris County. Their second role is to provide consultation and specialty care on a referral basis. In this role these hospitals are supportive of the consultative needs of local area hospitals and their medical staffs. The sources of referrals, however, extend far beyond Harris County to include much of the southern United States as well as Central and South America. Referral capacities are highly specialized and quite sophisticated. Finally, these institutions fulfill the important missions of medical education and academic research.

Three of these hospitals—Methodist, Texas Children's, and St. Luke's Episcopal—are exceptions to the downsizing of inpatient capacity that is otherwise the norm in the area. Expansions since 1983 include additional beds, outpatient facilities, and a new professional office building. Some construction continues at present. Hermann Hospital, however, was obliged to close 100 beds and to limit the scope of its emergency operation in order to maintain financial viability.

Multi-Institutional Systems. Multi-institutional systems have been the dominant organizational mode since the growth of for-profit enterprises in Harris County in the early 1970s. The more recent rise of not-for-profit chains in the area began about 1985. The Greater Houston Hospital Council estimates that 85 percent of its member organizations are now part of some type of multi-institutional system and that in the future this percentage will increase.

Large hospitals have initiated multi-institutional systems consisting of independent hospitals bound together by affiliation agreements or management contracts, but there is currently some decline in these kinds of arrangements. Two major hospitals in the Texas Medical Center, Methodist and Hermann, had developed extensive affiliations with large numbers of smaller hospitals in other cities, many in distant parts of Texas and in other states. In general, these affiliations were based on Methodist and Hermann offering services to smaller hospitals, such as hospital management services and consulting, in return for referral agreements. In recent years Hermann has divested itself of its Affiliated Systems subsidiary, and Methodist is said to be terminating many of its relationships. A reason cited by one hospital representative is that in the event of malpractice suits the "mother company" in a contractual agreement is likely to be included among those held liable by plaintiffs. It may also be speculated that the "feeder effect" of referrals from small hospitals to the "mother hospital" has not been sufficient to justify the affiliation.

Another multi-institutional form under some discussion locally is that of mergers. In 1989 two major hospitals briefly considered the possibility of merger, but nothing materialized. Some health care providers believe that mergers are inevitable, but there is no present evidence of pending actions. The consensus is that the usual mode of multi-institutional arrangements will continue to involve the ownership of hospitals by a corporate system, specific service-related affiliation agreements, participation in shared-service arrangements, and management contracts.

Hospital Financial Status. When interviews were conducted in early 1988, there was clear agreement that hospital economic fortunes were declining. In the second round of interviews in 1989, most observers believed that profit margins were continuing to drop, but a few thought the fiscal status of hospitals was improving as the economy improved. At the close of the study period, there was evidence that the profitability of most area hospitals was continuing to improve. Medicare cost reports for 1988 and earlier were obtained for ten major area hospitals. Seven reported operating income as a percentage of net revenue ranging from 6 to 22 percent for 1988, and all seven had higher operating incomes than in 1987. Of the other three hospitals, one showed an operating income of about 1 percent of net revenue, and the other two reported operating losses of approximately 2 percent and 5 percent of net revenue, respectively. These economic improvements occurred even though uncompensated care is said to continue to rise, perhaps reflecting the relatively large number of uninsured or underinsured people in the county despite the local economy's recovery.

Notwithstanding the positive experiences that have just been described, the pessimistic economic forecasts offered at the outset of this chapter have not changed. Careful management practices must be continued in light of the increasingly restrictive reimbursement policies. Although Medicare and Medicaid are identified as the most restrictive policies, private payers have also reduced payments, making it increasingly difficult for health care facilities to compensate for limited income from Medicare/Medicaid revenues by cost-shifting. The impact of revenue shortfalls or anticipated losses has resulted in several strategies:

- Increasing charges, either across the board or in selected services, for those who can pay for them.
- Developing alternative revenues by marketing outpatient surgery, imaging centers, or other services that can capture reimbursements outside of the DRG system. According to AHA reports, outpatient visits in Houston community hospitals increased by 69,700 between 1987 and 1988.
- Reducing expenses by laying off nonessential personnel in tandem with reducing the number of operating beds or by entering into management contracts or shared-service arrangements.
- Depleting reserves or endowment assets. (This option was described by only one observer and perhaps is not commonly pursued.)
- Supporting political action to persuade the U.S. Congress to increase federal third-party payments.

Three Houston-area hospitals closed in 1988-1989, including two small acute-care general hospitals and one rehabilitation/long-term-care facility. Both hospitals were small inner-city facilities patronized primarily by minority populations, a high percentage of whom were Medicaid patients. Interestingly, one of the inner-city hospitals and the long-term-care institution were both members of the same not-for-profit multi-institutional system. Closure of the inner-city hospitals was blamed by a spokesperson of the parent system on a drop-off in admissions and not on a preponderance of Medicaid patients. The same reason was given for closure of the rehabilitation/long-term-care hospital, which, in addition, suffered from a physical plant layout that was inefficient to maintain.

Physicians who had practiced in one of the inner-city hospitals that closed are making a major effort to find financing to reopen the facility. Although temporary financing was arranged with the multi-institutional system that had previously owned and operated it, a permanent solution could not be found and the hospital is defunct.

Emergency Medical and Trauma Care. At the outset of this study, many emergency rooms of varying capacity existed in Houston/Harris County, but only two emergency facilities had medical and surgical specialty support and back-up inpatient capacity to handle any type of emergency. These were both located in the Texas Medical Center about 200 yards apart. One was operated by Hermann Hospital and the other by the public hospital system at Ben Taub Hospital.

The emergency medical transportation system in Harris County is fragmented geographically. Houston's emergency transportation system is operated by the City of Houston Fire Department and is well staffed, trained, equipped, and supervised. The balance of the county, both the other municipalities and the unincorporated areas, is served by a patchwork of systems, with only a few on a par with Houston's. No countywide coordination exists at present, and no plans to develop such an emergency medical system are on the drawing boards.

In 1989 Hermann Hospital stopped accepting ambulance runs from the city's fire department. The principal reason given was that large numbers of individuals accepted for emergency care subsequently could not or would not pay their bills, and the hospital could not continue to absorb those losses. Consequently, there is now only one facility, the public hospital, that is capable of managing any medical or surgical emergency. Spokespersons for the Harris County Hospital District state that the public hospital can handle the increased load. Given the impact of emergency admissions on the district's inpatient capacity, described elsewhere in this chapter, it is uncertain how long the county's emergency needs can be met by one facility.

Outpatient and Non-acute Care. The dominant growth in health care facilities since 1984 has been in ambulatory-care facilities. At the same time that hospitals have in general, "down-sized" inpatient capacity, they have intensified and enhanced ambulatory services. The appeal continues to lie in the attraction of discretionary dollars, as hospitals compete successfully with other auspices of out-of-hospital services. This shift in emphasis is reflected not only in changing service locations but also in capital expenditures such as the construction of new or renovated outpatient facilities. Figures are not available, but one observer estimates that 90 percent of the capital outlay for area health care facilities from 1984 to 1989 was expended on outpatient facilities. Prior to 1984 about 80 percent or more of capital was invested in inpatient facilities. Outpatient surgery has especially flourished. One large hospital system reports that over 50 percent of its surgeries are currently performed in the ambulatory setting, up from 25 percent in 1986 and 15 percent in 1984.

Changes in psychiatric facilities run counter to the shift from inpatient to outpatient settings in general medical care. Growth of psychiatric hospital facilities in response to the increase in available reimbursement was described earlier. However, no discernible increase in psychiatric outpatient facilities has been noted. In fact, mental health care providers reported shortages in mental health halfway houses and day-care facilities.

There are two major rehabilitation hospitals of long standing experience in the Houston/Harris County area. They are the Texas Institute for Rehabilitation and Research, a not-for-profit, free-standing facility, and the Veterans Administration Medical Center. Both are part of the Texas Medical Center. Although other rehabilitation hospitals have not emerged in the Houston area, several new rehabilitation units have been established in acute-care general hospitals. As has been described, one hospital that provided both long-term nursing care and rehabilitation closed during the study period.

Outpatient psychiatric care is largely limited to office treatment provided by private practitioners on a fee-for-service or limited insurance basis and to public services offered by the Harris County Mental Health/ Mental Retardation Authority, a state-funded local service facility. A large number of voluntary agencies offer counseling of various sorts, funded in part by community contributions from the Gulf Coast United Way.

Impact of Prospective and Other Payment Systems. Reimbursement based on diagnosis-related groups has contributed to the closure of small institutions or, at the least, has stressed their economic balance severely. Larger institutions have survived this change in reimbursement policy and are financially improved, some slightly and several significantly. Two results of the policy shift have been shortened lengths of hospital stay and reductions in number of beds. Diversification of facilities has been stimulated so that care can be offered outside the inpatient setting, for example, through ambulatory and home care. Such diversification has permitted the provision of care in less expensive environments and has allowed hospitals to seek other revenue sources. Finally, many believe that shorter lengths of stay have resulted in the discharge of patients who are sicker than their counterparts in earlier days of longer hospital stays.

In commenting on the general atmosphere in health care, one physician expressed concern that the relationship between patients, physicians, and hospitals is becoming markedly adversarial as insurance companies and the Health Care Financing Administration reduce coverage. A widely held variation on this view is that the instigation of diagnosis-related reimbursement brought hospitals and physicians closer together in dealing with the economic limits imposed by the payment system. Increasingly, both consumers and providers of health care suffer greater financial risk. No one believes these restrictions have had any favorable impact on the cost of care because expenditures continue to rise.

The role of state government in financing public systems of care for the indigent continues to grow. State expenditures increase, and county governments must assume greater responsibility in financing indigent care. Recently enacted state laws have authorized increased participation in Medicaid, grants-in-aid for high-risk maternity patients ineligible for Medicaid, and grants-in-aid for primary health care demonstrations. Today each county must assume the costs of care for a limited number of indigent county residents who are categorically ineligible for Medicaid but have income levels that match Medicaid-eligibility requirements. More detail is provided about state and federal programs for the poor in the discussion of access to care.

Because of state financing, some level of payment is available to hospitals for patients who would otherwise pay nothing for their care. Hospital representatives point out, however, that this financial relief is inadequate because the reimbursement levels are below costs and the opportunity to shift cost deficits to paying patients is diminishing. In fact, in some parts of Texas, it is exceedingly difficult to find providers willing to participate in the state's expanded maternity care program. However, as a result of expanded Medicaid eligibility, a higher proportion of indigent women are likely to have prenatal care during their pregnancies, which should lead to fewer babies born with low birth weights or other complications and should reduce requirements for neonatal intensive care admissions.

Unabated increases in health insurance premiums continue in Harris County. Although benefit packages are somewhat broader—for example, including dental care and psychiatric care—the insured are being placed more at risk, either by employers or by insurers. Deductibles and copayments are increasing. Incentives in the form of lower copayments are offered those who opt for providers that discount or participate in health promotion programs or managed-care arrangements. Some small firms are dropping insurance as an employee benefit altogether; others are employing a higher proportion of workers on contract or other classifications with no fringe benefits.

As Medicare eliminates the pass-through reimbursement for teaching costs, academic medical centers are forced to look elsewhere for financing. One center developed an active fee-for-service private practice option. Although this solution has reduced the supply of teaching patients and has limited faculty teaching time, it has allowed faculty to develop teaching models in practice settings and is proving an effective method for revenue generation.

Alternative Delivery Systems. Alternative delivery systems became major options for care in the 1980s in Harris County. Two features characterize such systems: changes in financing and pricing (prepayment and discounting) and care settings that are alternatives to inpatient facilities. Alternative delivery systems include health maintenance organizations, preferred provider organizations, ambulatory care offices in shopping malls (urgi-centers), ambulatory surgery centers, and free-standing diagnostic facilities typified by imaging centers. In the latter, sophisticated imaging equipment such as the computerized tomographic scanner and the nuclear magnetic resonator are available, devices that were housed only in hospitals when they first became available. Changes in the organization and service offerings of physician office practices have accompanied the introduction of alternative delivery systems, and in many instances, office practices have been linked to the alternative systems—that is, through independent practice associations, health maintenance organizations, and/or preferred provider organizations.

Increasingly restrictive reimbursement policies in public medical care financing programs and private health insurance, plus strategies and practices of major corporations in the interest of health care cost containment, have proven to be the most powerful stimuli for the development of alternative systems and for subsequent changes in these systems. Many of the latter have been mediated through the Houston Area Health Care Coalition, an organization of local corporate interests. These pressures have stimulated the growth of alternative financing mechanisms, both prepayment and discounted fees. The growth of outpatient and other care settings has been abetted by the belief that such facilities will result in less costly health and medical care. The maintenance of adequate volumes of patients and cash flow have proven to be strong incentives for physicians and hospitals to become involved with alternative delivery systems. Most hospitals in Harris County have an affiliation with either a health maintenance organization or a preferred provider organization or both. About 8 percent of all hospital admissions are HMO- or PPO-affiliated patients.

In this dynamic milieu, dramatic changes have occurred in the status of individual alternative delivery systems, even within the short period of this study. At the outset of the inquiry (1987), health maintenance organizations were prominent in the area. After a decade of growth they were at the height of development, both in numbers of organizations and in total enrollments. Opinion among those interviewed, however, was almost evenly divided concerning the continuing strength of HMOs in the county. Those who were optimistic spoke about recent facility expansions locally and forecasted a new period of growth in enrollments. An equal number pointed to a leveling in these same statistics and to dissatisfaction among business sponsors and individual users and predicted a decline in the prepaid industry. Events at the end of the 1980s have borne out the predictions of the latter.

In 1987 most hospitals had some kind of contractual relationship with HMOs. By the study's end, HMOs had plateaued and hospitals were less interested in contractual relationships with them; rather, negotiations were proceeding with preferred provider organizations or directly with industry. Enrollment statistics reflected a shift of approximately equal numbers of corporate users from HMOs to PPOs. Current predictions of several of those interviewed are that this eminence of PPOs will also give way to direct negotiations for managed-care arrangements between corporate organizations and hospital and group practice systems. This trend appears to be a movement away from a reliance on intermediate organizations as agents negotiating and organizing the encounters between payers and providers.

Hospital Sponsorship of Alternative Systems. According to those interviewed, the sponsorship of alternative delivery systems by hospitals accelerated during the study period. This trend has occurred at the expense of free-standing alternative systems and facilities, as hospitals have competed successfully for sponsorship of these new alternatives with independent entrepreneurs. The prime example of hospital success is in the case of ambulatory surgery.

Ambulatory surgery centers continue to thrive in Harris County. As these surgi-centers developed, they were owned and operated by physicians or free-standing corporations that negotiated with hospitals for back-up inpatient care and other services. At present, the hospitals themselves are competing successfully as the owners and operators of these centers. The concept of ambulatory surgery is viable and acceptable to providers and to consumers. Hospitals find them to be good alternative revenue sources and are in a favorable position to compete with other sponsors.

The number of urgi-centers, or "Docs-in-the-Box," as they have been dubbed, has declined dramatically in Harris County in recent years. This decline is thought to be related to competition from the resurgence of hospital emergency room walk-in business, which is now being advertised, organized and priced like ambulatory primary care centers.

Physician Office Practice. Several observations emerged from the study regarding the status of physician office practice as it relates to alternative delivery systems. Physician office practice may be thought of as a traditional, rather than an alternative, delivery system. The development of HMOs, PPOs, and hospital-sponsored outpatient services may be perceived as a threat to the income of office practitioners if not to office practice itself. Physicians, especially those in group practices, seem to have successfully organized to compete. One factor in this success would appear to be the physicians' ability to organize themselves in their present settings to offer prepayment or discounted service arrangements, either as providers for HMOs or PPOs or on their own. At the same time, they have continued to offer traditional fee-for-service practice.

Another competitive advantage is the ability of physicians in office practice to offer the same wide range of procedures that have typified alternative systems. They are able to provide services once performed in the more expensive hospital setting and thereby satisfy demands of insurers and business. Examples of the range of procedures offered in physicians' offices include endoscopies, ambulatory and minor surgeries (including cataract surgery), ultrasound, stress tests, noninvasive cardiac diagnostic procedures, imaging, nuclear medicine, and infusion therapy. The strategy of physician involvement in joint ventures with hospitals is relatively uncommon in Harris County.

The Impact of Alternative Delivery Systems on Health Care in Houston/Harris County. Alternative delivery systems are at present important players in the Houston area. It is estimated that the total combined enrollment of salaried persons in area HMOs and PPOs was approximately 8 percent of the labor force, just under 1.5 million, in 1989. Even if more direct health care contracts between businesses and large providers are negotiated and intermediary systems bypassed, the market for HMOs and PPOs organized separately from hospital or corporate structures probably will not be altogether eliminated. Many businesses and providers are simply not large enough to organize alternative systems without a third party. Moreover, prepayment and discounting have become accepted practices, as has been the use of ambulatory settings for services and procedures previously limited to inpatient settings. In summary, although there probably will be a shift in the sponsorship of alternative systems to hospitals and, perhaps, to physician groups, HMOs and PPOs will continue to have an active role in the financing and delivery of health and medical care in the region.

Summary of Principal Changes in the Acute-Care System. There were surprising changes during the short monitoring period in the several components of the acute-care system. By the end of the decade, hospitals had achieved greater diversification of service delivery, successful entry into the alternative care market, down-sizing of inpatient facilities, and improvement in profitability. Similarly, physician office practices were emerging as successful competitors in the sponsorship of alternative delivery systems. Health maintenance organizations and preferred provider organizations battled it out during the decade for a small but significant sector of the market, with PPOs winning out as the study ended. The principal pressures for these changes were restrictive reimbursement for inpatient services and corporate interest in less costly service sites for their insured employees.

Emergency medical care and transportation systems worsened during the study period. Emergency systems outside the city of Houston were fragmented and uneven in quality and support. This situation did not improve during the decade, and no systematic efforts to plan or establish a countywide system were identified. The system that served the emergency patients inside city limits declined in capacity as one of the two major trauma centers found difficulty in covering its financial expenses with revenues from patients receiving emergency care. The hospital stopped accepting emergency ambulance runs from the City of Houston Fire Department.

The Long-Term Care System

In contrast to what had occurred in the acute-care system, there was very little change in the long-term-care system. The incentives and disincentives for the development and operation of long-term-care services remained the same throughout the 1980s.

Long-term-care options in the Houston community include home care, nursing homes, limited day care, and a few hospices. One new entrepreneurial venture offers transitional care, a level of contractual service offered to health maintenance organizations and other managed-care arrangements. High-quality, intensive nursing is provided in a nonhospital facility as an appropriate means of intermediate care between hospital and home care. The service insures convalescent care at a less expensive rate than that provided by hospitals. Most readily available of all of the aforementioned options are nursing homes and home care.

The largest proportion of nursing homes are for-profit ventures, which reflects a long-standing move in Texas away from not-for-profit ownership. Growth of these institutions in the state has been indolent, about 3 to 4 percent each year. The payment source for about 95 percent of nursing home patients is Medicaid. The Texas Department of Human Services, which administers the Medicaid program, sets the reimbursement rate prospectively.

Given this slow growth rate, the number of beds and facilities has been relatively stable, and there has been little development of new types of facilities or new ownership types. Nevertheless, some small innovations in nursing home care have been introduced, for example, facilities for ventilator-assisted patients.

Home care is offered by the traditional not-for-profit Visiting Nurses Association (VNA) and by a large number of for-profit enterprises, many of which are operated by hospitals. Home care agencies experienced rapid growth from 1982 to 1985, largely in response to federal regulatory revisions granting for-profit agencies eligibility for Medicare reimbursement. Hospitals participated actively in developing their own home care services as part of this growth. The Visiting Nurse Association, the largest home care agency, has survived an economic crisis posed by the appearance of competitive for-profit agencies. The VNA includes in its services a special home care project for AIDS patients.

The incentive for hospital involvement in home care is twofold: (1) the pressure of diagnosis-related group reimbursement for earlier discharge, increasing the need for after-care for patients who leave the hospital early; and (2) the previously mentioned changes in Medicare that made for-profit systems eligible for reimbursement and provided hospitals that developed home care agencies with additional options for revenue. Hospitals can claim after-care reimbursement, which covers the cost of convalescent care, and can thereby avoid the limitations that the prospective payment system places on inpatient care had those patients not been discharged. Despite these incentives, several hospital representatives noted that many hospitals are getting out of the home care business and referring discharged patients to other home care agencies. Perhaps the operation of their own agencies has not proven as profitable as the hospitals had anticipated.

Hospices are just now becoming popular in Harris County. No large ones have been constructed; the normal accommodation is six to ten patients or fewer. Limitations appear to be those of inadequate reimbursement. There is very limited hospice capacity in two facilities attempting to meet the needs of AIDS patients. One day-care facility for AIDS patients began operation during the study period. Acquired by the public hospital system, it is a renovated general hospital, now operated for the care of indigent patients.

Formal links between the acute-care and long-term-care systems are found in the discharge planning of private hospitals that operate home care services and in at least one large state university hospital with an active discharge-planning service. To date, no systematic planning activity has attempted to define long-term-care needs on a population basis and to match these needs with existing resources and/or barriers to access.

The inability of individuals to pay for long-term care and the inadequate reimbursement levels of current financing programs have been major problems in the adequate provision of these services. In addition, no long-term-care facilities exist for psychiatric patients. There has been some discussion in the state legislature and among policymakers at conferences about insurance and other plans to address this problem. Most express the view that private insurance alone cannot cover the financial requirements. No definitive legislative proposals for public solutions have been offered thus far.

One solution to both the problem of too few long-term, skilled-care beds and that of the closure of small hospitals is the "swing bed" concept. Certain beds in a hospital are designated for both acute-hospital-care use and skilled-care use. They can be switched back and forth in response to needs and thus improve the likelihood that the facility will maintain better occupancy levels and improved financial viability.

Media interest in long-term care has been expressed in two areas: (1) as part of the more general problem of the lack of availability of services for AIDS patients, and (2) in discussions of the recurrent failures of some nursing homes to maintain minimum standards of care established by state regulatory agencies. The system is plagued by complaints and occasional documentation of poor quality. Newspaper accounts of violations of Texas Department of Health regulations are not uncommon.

The Public Sector

Although the majority of health care encounters occur in the private sector, the public sector is, nevertheless, heavily utilized. The large numbers of indigent, uninsured, and underinsured persons in Harris County stress the capacity of the public health agencies and the hospital district. As has been noted, the numbers of vulnerable people are both large and increasing.

Public Hospitals

The public hospital responsibility is fulfilled by a county entity, the Harris County Hospital District. The management of the hospital district is the responsibility of a seven-member board of managers appointed by the Harris County Commissioners Court, the county's governing body. The statutory responsibility of the Hospital District is to provide medical care for the poor of the county. It has just completed the construction of two new hospitals, which are replacements for existing hospitals that are now closed to patient care. These new facilities were opened during the later stages of the study.

The district is a large, comprehensive complex of two major hospitals, one smaller hospital, a newly acquired day facility for AIDS patients, and a network of ten neighborhood health centers that provide ambulatory care. A total of 1,043 beds is provided in the three hospitals, representing a net increase of almost 300 beds over the combined capacity of the two recently replaced hospitals. The district's annual operating budget exceeds $250 million. In the fiscal year ending March 31, 1989, the district's hospitals admitted approximately 55,000 inpatients. Of this group 31.5 percent were obstetrical patients, 27.5 percent newborns, 34.4 percent medical and surgical, and 6.7 percent other pediatric patients. In the same period neighborhood clinics cared for 190,783 individuals, by unduplicated count.

The financing of the hospital district is derived from multiple sources, of which the largest is an ad valorem property tax, accounting for approximately 70 percent of revenues. Other sources include Medicaid, Medicare, patient fees, and auxiliary services such as parking. There is no expressed interest by county elected officials in the "privatization" of either the public hospital system or the county public health department. The Houston Department of Health and Human Services (DHHS), however, is developing an initiative that is expected to result in private operators contracting with the city to provide public health services in a clinic to be developed in the southwest part of the city.

Eligibility for care in the Harris County Hospital District is based on residency in the county and limited income. The hospital district has a sliding scale, in which patients at the lowest levels of income pay nothing. The proportion of the bill for which patients are responsible increases as their income does. Approximately 750,000 persons are eligible for care among the total population of just under three million. According to patient origin studies, most patients who use district facilities live within the central city. That area has traditionally consisted of low-income neighborhoods. The district's facilities are located in proximity to most of Harris County's indigent population. In recent years, however, pockets of poverty have developed in many other quarters of the city and county that had previously been populated only by nonindigent families.

During Houston's recent economic downturn, the district began seeing patients who were newly poor and who had never before used public facilities. Many of these individuals have returned to work, but because employment conditions leave substantial numbers of people uninsured or underinsured, some workers continue to seek care at public facilities. The district's chief executive officer stated that in 1985, 11,000 patients were new to the district. By 1990 that figure was estimated to reach 37,000.

The proportion of Hispanic users of district services has been steadily rising in recent years. A high proportion have low incomes. Another new group is made up of the homeless. Houston newspapers estimate this population to be between 10,000 and 35, 000. Families are thought to constitute 40 percent of this group. Recently the hospital district, with a federal grant of approximately $1 million, initiated health care delivery at homeless shelters.

There are varying perceptions of the quality of care provided by the hospital district. On the one hand, quality of care is good because it is provided by the faculty and staff of the two medical schools, who offer a high level of supervision. On the other hand, overcrowding of patients stresses the system. Given the large number of people eligible for care and the relatively small number of beds, disproportionately large amounts of resources are devoted to emergency or otherwise delayed and serious admissions. Elective or timely admissions are crowded out.

The chief executive officer stated his belief that for much of the 1990s the Harris County Hospital District will continue to serve as the medical care safety net for the indigent and those "caught in the middle." The district will likely move in the direction of facilitating or directly providing public health preventive services, such as prenatal care, that should reduce the demand for inpatient services. Another strategy will involve the improvement of revenue flow from other sources in order to reduce the district's dependency on the local property tax.

The Public Health System

The major providers of public health services in Harris County are two local governmental entities, the Harris County Health Department and the Houston Department of Health and Human Services (DHHS). Other public health responsibilities are borne by separate departments or units of local government. Air and water quality control outside the Houston city limits is enforced not by the county health department but by a separate department of county government. Protection from arthropod-borne disease is provided by the Harris County Mosquito Control District, also a separate county entity. Publicly financed mental health/mental retardation services are made available by the Harris County Mental Health/ Mental Retardation Authority, a state-financed institution, and by voluntary agencies, many of which are funded by the Gulf Coast United Way. School health services are the responsibility of twenty-three independent school districts within the county.

Above the local level are state agencies, federal agencies, and a tricounty quasi-public entity that treats industrial waste on a fee-for-service basis. State and federal agencies offer regulatory protection against exposure to industrial and environmental hazards.

The Houston DHHS, by far the larger of the two public health agencies, had more than 1,000 employees and a budget of just over $30 million in FY 1989. In contrast, the Harris County Health Department had a budget of $8 million and employed approximately 270 persons. The county health department budget and staff from 1987 to 1989 were stable. The budget rose steadily from $5.5 million in 1984 to $8 million in 1987. At that time, the city health department was coping with drastic reductions in its budget that were imposed earlier as tax revenues declined in the economic downturn. In FY 1988 those cuts were restored, and in the following year, the department was rehiring.

Primary financial support for the two health departments is the ad valorem property tax. The city captures federal grants-in-aid directly, whereas the county receives a smaller proportion of its budget from this source. Federal money makes up about 28 percent of the county public health budget; most of the federal dollars are passed through the state health department. Other sources of revenue for the two departments include Medicaid reimbursements in selected programs and patient fees. The latter are small and do not cover the cost of services, but they constitute in the aggregate a significant level of revenue.

The program of the city health department is broader than that of the county, which is in accord with its larger budget and staff. For example, the city is involved in several central administrative programs and some public health programs that are not part of the responsibility of the county health department. In the former category are city vital statistics registration and a health planning program. County vital events are registered not by the county health department but by the Harris County clerk.

In the area of public health, the city administers large air and water quality control programs and an occupational health program, it operates a public health laboratory, it is responsible—along with the fire department—for part of the city's emergency medical system, and it provides health services at the city jail. In addition, in the mid-1980s community development and other social programs of the city were added to the responsibilities of the city health department. The two components of the Houston DHHS, health and human services, are administered separately.

The county health department also differs from the city in that it has fairly large programs for the education of water treatment plant operators as well as programs for the inspection of these plants and of septic tanks in the extensive suburban/rural area in its jurisdiction.

The city and county departments share in common responsibility for the traditional public health programs, including epidemiologic surveillance and analysis, maternal and child health services, communicable disease control, immunizations, family planning, dental health, health education, chronic disease control, the Women, Infant and Children's (WIC) nutritional program, animal control, general sanitation (including food protection services), and abatement of nuisances. These programs are administered by the two departments in their respective jurisdictions with little or no duplication of service populations.

The city health department is the recipient of a large federal grant for AIDS, some of which is subcontracted to several community-based organizations. The health department has been heavily criticized in the local media for its handling of the AIDS funding. The federal government has been critical of public and private AIDS care providers in Houston, generally, for their inability to coordinate services, and as a result, the awarding of federal funds to Houston has been delayed. By the end of the study period there were signs that this situation was improving and that money and services were beginning to flow more smoothly.

Major public health concerns are AIDS, immunizations, and maternal and child health. A growing concern is the problem of exposure to toxic substances, both in the ambient population and in the workplace. Maternal and child health concerns center around a drop in the use of prenatal care that coincided with reductions in service as the result of budget cuts. Measles is the primary immunization issue. In the late 1980s the city experienced a measles epidemic, which appeared to be nearing its end as the study ended.

The Health Professions Work Force

The observations that have been reported thus far relate to the systems of private and public care in Houston and Harris County. The adequacy and effectiveness of those systems are dependent on the professionals who provide and administer services. The two key professions are physicians and nurses.

Physician Supply

There is divided opinion and evidence regarding the presence or absence of a physician surplus. Studies of the numbers of physicians in the state show a dramatic slowing in the rate of increase during the 1980s. This deceleration is primarily due to two factors: (1) in-migration of doctors trained in other states has lessened, and (2) changes in state licensure requirements have reduced the number of foreign medical graduates entering practice. The relative ease of recruiting physicians, reported by representatives of public health departments and HMOs, provides anecdotal evidence in support of the contention that there is an oversupply of physicians. Some observers point out, however, that although there are larger numbers of physicians available than in the past, there has been a reduction in physicians' productivity, that is, the number of hours per week they are willing to work. The physician that has been in practice for many years is accustomed to work weeks of more than seventy hours, whereas younger physicians are seeking careers that allow more time for family and other activities. A second factor is the increasing proportion of women attending medical school. In 1987, for example, 50 percent of the entering class of one local school were women. It is expected that female physicians will spend less time in practice than male physicians because they also fulfill maternal roles.

Opinions about relative surpluses and shortages vary by specialty. Some believe there is an oversupply of general surgeons, psychiatrists, anesthesiologists, chest surgeons, plastic surgeons, and radiologists. According to one observer, oversupply of anesthesiologists has limited the market for nurse anesthetists. In short supply are child psychiatrists and obstetricians; the latter shortage is probably related to professional liability risk, which is rated higher in obstetrics than in many other specialties.

Although most local observers acknowledge that the present physician supply is plentiful (with the exception of the two specialties just cited), the current physician surplus in Texas is not seen as a problem requiring correction. Even physicians, who themselves might be expected to worry about the competitive aspects of oversupply, do not appear to be concerned.

Nurse Supply

In 1987 there was a significant shortage of hospital nurses. Many reasons were given: inadequate compensation relative to responsibility and amount of work, uninteresting jobs, failure to be given more "say" about decisions, and undesirable working hours, among others. The shortage was primarily in hospitals, long-term-care facilities, and health departments. No shortage of nurses, however, existed in psychiatric hospitals, where the job was said to be more prestigious, or in school health systems, perhaps a reflection of better working hours and salaries. A nursing shortage was present, but not as severe, in office practice.

Efforts to remedy the nursing shortage were as numerous as the reasons for the shortages. The efforts included recruiting in foreign countries, increasing salaries, introducing profit-sharing schemes, enhancing the job content and prestige, and adopting a variety of flex-time and part-time arrangements.

As the study period came to a close, informants generally agreed that although the availability of nurses continued to be a problem, the nursing shortage was easing, except in rural areas of Harris County and in long-term care facilities. Most thought that efforts to increase salaries and improve working conditions had helped. Decreases in operating beds also somewhat reduced the demand for nurses. These factors are consistent with recent national and regional studies of nurse supply and demand.

Professional School Enrollments

The health professional schools in Harris County have not pursued consistent policies with respect to class size. Starting in 1981 dental schools in Texas, including that of The University of Texas Health Science Center at Houston, have voluntarily reduced the number of their entering students in response to intense lobbying of Texas legislators by the state dental association. The association perceived an oversupply of practicing dentists in Texas. In schools of medicine, nursing, and allied health, class sizes had not changed appreciably as late as 1990, nor had professional associations pressured for change.

Applications to medical schools have declined in Houston as elsewhere. The size of entering classes of nurses has not changed, although recent reports indicate that numbers of applications are increasing.

Access to Care

The changes in the population, the economy, the health care system, and reimbursement have affected the accessibility of care to vulnerable populations. The following sections address the state of those populations, changes in Medicaid reimbursement, and various state initiatives.

Insured, Underinsured and Uninsured Populations

Self- or company-insured individuals can gain ready access to private sector care in Houston. Outpatient and ambulatory surgery treatments sponsored by hospitals are also available, as is home care, especially high-tech procedures such as intravenous infusion therapy.

Insurance benefit trends, however, compromise the financial accessibility of these services to increasing proportions of the insured. With each new health insurance contract period, higher deductibles and copayments increase out-of-pocket expenses. The minimum income necessary to support adequate insurance is going up. Each year a larger number of employed persons are thereby becoming underinsured.

For Harris county as a whole, the declining number of hospital beds has not affected access to hospital care because inpatient utilization has also declined, albeit slightly. As noted earlier, this decline reflects a shift in utilization to outpatient and home-care settings. Although most hospitals have closed some beds and a few have shut their doors altogether, the number of licensed beds has remained constant.

The number of uninsured residents in Harris County increased during the economic downturn, which reached its low point in 1986-1987. As people found jobs in the recovery that followed, there was a resurgence in the number of persons insured, but not to the same level of coverage. Many employers had reduced coverage or discontinued health insurance as an employment benefit altogether. Many new hires were classified as hourly wage earners on contracts without fringe benefits. Although there are no figures to document with precision the number of uninsured or underinsured, public hospital officials report large numbers of care-seekers who previously had been insured. The interview panel for this study also generally confirmed this decline in the insured population.

Access to care for some categories of uninsured populations improved modestly during the study period. Factors principally responsible were the economic recovery, expansions of Medicaid eligibility for maternal and child health services, and various state and federal grant-in-aid programs. The homeless, for example, now have a federally financed ambulatory-care project administered by the public hospital system. Health services are provided in homeless shelters operated by the city of Houston.

Significant numbers of uninsured individuals rely on the Harris County Hospital District as their only available health care source; others show up as uncompensated-care patients in private hospitals. Major categories of the uninsured and underinsured include minority populations, who are overrepresented among the indigent; many of the elderly; and the homeless and refugee populations. The ethnic makeup of the indigent population in Harris County reflects increasing numbers of Hispanics, whereas the number of blacks has remained stable.

The Medicaid Population

The number of area Medicaid recipients increased during the study period, due primarily to state participation in several Medicaid-coverage expansions. Pregnant women without children, presumed to be Medicaid-eligible at delivery, became eligible for maternity and infant care. Pregnant women living with their husbands but with sufficiently low family income also became eligible for Medicaid benefits, as did their children. Income eligibility increased to 130 percent of poverty for pregnant women and infants and to 100 percent of poverty for children up to age four in FY 1989 and to age six in FY 1990.

Evidence of increased use of prenatal and intrapartum care was demonstrated in a neighboring county clinic that accepts Medicaid reimbursement. Staff there reported a significant increase in the percentage of Medicaid patients since these expansions were enacted.

The majority of the nonmaternity indigent population of Texas nevertheless remain ineligible for Medicaid because of the income ceiling mandated by the state, which is slightly greater than one third of the federally defined poverty level. The eligibility screening process, despite efforts to streamline it, remains cumbersome. Many who would be eligible do not complete this process and do not become recipients. Consequently, less than one half of the state's indigent population, as defined by federal guidelines, are eligible for Medicaid, and fewer than that number actually go through the qualifying process. In Harris County a greater proportion of the poor than in the state has access to care because the public hospital system serves indigents up to and above the federal poverty norm on a sliding payment scale based on income and family size.

There are significant limitations in access to medical care for Medicaid patients in the Houston area. Most private physicians do not accept them. Reasons stated include inadequate and delayed reimbursements. Physicians—often minority members—with offices in low-income neighborhoods are the exceptions; they usually accept Medicaid patients.

Most hospitals will admit Medicaid recipients, but the payer mix varies considerably by hospital. Medicare cost reports for 1988 were obtained for ten hospitals. Of these, eight hospitals showed that Medicaid discharges as a percentage of total discharges ranged from zero to approximately 20 percent. Two of these hospitals, both investor-owned facilities, reported no Medicaid patients among their discharges for that year.

The 1988 payer mix of Medicaid patients in Harris County hospitals overall was 6 percent. This figure is influenced by the presence of the public hospital system to which providers as a rule refer Medicaid patients. Without the public system the average Medicaid and uncompensated-care load might be higher. The other principal reason cited for the limitation of Medicaid admissions is that reimbursements are considered to fall below actual costs. Too high a proportion of Medicaid and/or Medicare patients is considered an economic liability to the hospital.

The Harris County Hospital District readily accepts Medicaid and Medicare reimbursement. The Houston Health Department serves Medicaid-eligible patients in its prenatal care clinics. Medicaid is the dominant payer of nursing home care, covering approximately 95 percent of nursing home patients.

The Local Impacts of State Initiatives

In the mid-1980s, state participation in indigent health care increased formally. The total amount of new expenditures in authorizing legislation was not large—approximately $300 million per year—but it was nevertheless significant. Several new statutes were introduced, the most important of which were programs to expand Medicaid eligibility for maternal and child care; to finance maternity care for indigent women ineligible for Medicaid; to set up primary care demonstration programs for the indigent; and to mandate the responsibility of each county to assure medical care for non-Medicaid-covered indigents up to 10 percent of the county's yearly tax revenues. The latter statute does not affect Harris County because of the preexisting hospital district. These programs survived the last legislative session that was held during the study period. In fact, legislators modestly increased benefits.

Historically, access to health and medical care has been viewed in Harris County as a local and federal responsibility. This view is reflected in the willingness of local government to levy taxes for this purpose and in the Medicaid program of the federal government. A current effort to "get more bang for the federal buck" is manifest in attempts to gain a better match of federal Medicaid dollars with local and state dollars already being spent. In recent years, as the Texas legislature has enacted state-financed health care programs, public providers in Harris County have added those resources to their efforts. Whether these state initiatives represent a growing trend of state responsibility in the care of the indigent remains to be seen.

The Harris County Hospital District's capacity continues to be stressed by the growth of the uninsured population, notwithstanding the 300-bed increase in the system. This situation is compounded by the fact that the district is now the primary provider of emergency care in the county. Thus, not only is a heavy burden saddled onto the emergency facility, but also other less urgent and elective admissions to the public hospital are often delayed.

The news media have devoted attention to the problems of access to health and medical care of Harris County's homeless, but inadequate health care has been treated as only one aspect of the plight of the homeless rather than as a primary issue for discussion. According to newspaper estimates, 10,000 to 30,000 homeless people, of whom 40 percent are families, wander the streets of Houston. Judging from the amount of space accorded the subject, access to adequate health care by the indigent per se is not a significant media issue.

Public Policy

Health matters have not been among the issues that politicians live or die by in their election campaigns. They have been of sufficient importance, however, that considerable legislative action occurs. In Texas, substantive health legislation as a proportion of all enactments has increased steadily since the early 1970s. Often action is the result of federal legislation that requires state participation, such as Medicaid or the National Health Planning and Resources Development Act of 1974. Increasingly, however, the state has addressed health issues on its own initiative.

Local and state groups, professional associations, and agencies have been instrumental in pressuring government to establish, review, and/or change state health policy. Groups that have been active advocates of recent legislation include the March of Dimes Birth Defects Foundation, the Healthy Mothers/Healthy Babies Coalition, the Texas Human Services Foundation, the Children's Defense Fund, the Texas Medical Association, the Texas Hospital Association, the Texas Public Health Association, various AIDS providers, the Texas Department of Human Services, and the Texas Department of Health. Each of these has representation in Harris County.

Legislative Action

The Texas legislature meets every two years, the latest regular session during the study period having been in 1989. The most significant health-related legislation enacted in that session pertained to AIDS and indigent health care. Other issues addressed included hospice care, workers' compensation, rural health, and United States–Mexico border health issues.

For FY 1990 and FY 1991 the legislature appropriated $7.9 million and $10.5 million, respectively, for AIDS education and service. These amounts represented approximately a fivefold increase over previous levels of state funding. The major part of these appropriations were to the Texas Department of Health, which was directed to use them to complement available federal funding. About $1.0 million was also appropriated to two University of Texas institutions to establish AIDS-related research units.

Other legislation designated the Texas Commission on Alcohol and Drug Abuse as the lead agency for issues relating to substance abusers who have, or are at risk of, HIV infection. The commission was instructed to develop, along with other appropriate agencies, a plan outlining needs and delineating each agency's role and responsibility for counseling and testing, for residential and outpatient treatment for substance abusers, for community outreach programs, and for staff training. The Texas Department of Human Services is charged with conducting a comprehensive study of the availability of foster care and day-care services for HIV-infected children and evaluating the availability of services for families in which more than one member is infected with HIV.

In addition to the Medicaid expansions described earlier, the enacted legislation restored provider reimbursement reductions, amounting up to

4.5 percent made in 1986. Other legislation directed selected hospital districts and teaching hospitals to transfer funds to the state's Disproportionate Share Fund, the money from which is distributed to hospitals providing the greatest amounts of indigent health care. The money transferred to the fund is matched with federal funds and thus results in increases in funding available to the state for health care services to the poor.

The Maternal and Infant Health Improvement Act and the Primary Care Act, cornerstones of the state's indigent health care initiative, were continued with slight increases in appropriations. Another enactment established an insurance pool for persons who are either uninsurable or afflicted by medical conditions that place them in an extremely high-cost health insurance category. Persons in this pool pay limited premiums. Funded by premiums, the pool assesses a fee on all companies providing health insurance in Texas. If costs exceed revenues, these insurance companies are then eligible for fee-reimbursement by the state in the next fiscal cycle.

Other legislation enacted in 1989 authorized the Texas Department of Health to establish licensing procedures for facilities providing nursing or medical care to persons with AIDS or other terminal illnesses. In addition, the Texas Department of Human Services was directed to establish demonstration projects in nursing facilities to assess the costs of providing care to HIV-infected people, to demonstrate the need for specialized long-term nursing care, and to provide teaching programs on caring for people with HIV infection.

An omnibus bill was enacted with provisions, among many others, to provide relief for small rural hospitals. Although major financing was not included, an Office of Rural Health was established in the Texas Department of Health. Also, because of growing local, state, and federal interest in issues of health and economic development along the Mexico–United States border, another office in the state health department was established to monitor border health events and perform planning functions.

Legislation was enacted in response to increasing the loss of coverage due to the escalation of premiums and court settlements in recent years. In Harris County 7.6 percent of the patient mix by payer in 1988 was accounted for by patients insured under that program. The legislation made no major changes in insurance premiums or structure but established a commission to oversee a more stringent effort to eliminate perceived abuses in the system.

State Health Planning and Certificate of Need

The Statewide Health Coordinating Council (SHCC), housed in and staffed by the Texas Department of Health, is the lone Texas remnant of the National Health Planning and Resources Development Act of 1974.

Every two years the SHCC publishes a state health plan. The most recent plan identified thirteen priority health issues and enumerated regional priorities in the twenty-four state planning regions. Distributed widely, the plan is used as a major source of information by legislators and others. Neither the plan nor the planning process is otherwise formally tied into the policy-making structure of the state. There is no certificate-of-need program. It was repealed in 1983, when the state was first given that option by Congress.

Unresolved Health Policy Issues

The state of Texas is not as active as some other states in addressing issues of health care cost containment in the private sector or assuring financial access to care, other than for the indigent population. In the latter arena, however, there was more legislative energy expended in the 1980s than in previous years. In general, the legislative philosophy is an antiregulatory one. Regulatory interventions are usually undertaken only if there is a perception of imminent federal regulation, either by statute or by court action (and state action is seen as the only means to circumvent federal intervention), or if there is a perception that serious economic consequences will result from the state's failure to intervene as regulator.

In the course of the present investigation, local health care providers and consumers made the following recommendations concerning issues that they felt merited increased governmental attention:

- There should be a well-articulated national health policy; the absence of such a clear policy was seen as a severe hindrance in the rational delivery of quality care.
- Minimum health insurance coverage should be mandated by the state.
- Long-term-care financing should be increased.
- The government should take over the responsibility for the provision of adequate care that has been saddled upon the backs of providers; it does not make sense to reimburse less than costs.
- The ethical and practical issues related to the rationing of health care should be seriously considered.
- Nurses should be given increased responsibility for patient care.
- There should be state support for systematic long-range planning.

Summary and Principal Observations

Perhaps the most impressive finding that has emerged from the study of events during the 1987-1989 period and the entire decade of the 1980s is the number of rapid changes that occurred. Over the decade there were significant shifts in the distribution and makeup of the population. Substantial numbers of Anglo residents moved out of the city into the county, and a diverse cultural mix of blacks, Hispanics, Anglos, and Asians developed. The economy dipped dramatically and then recovered in a few short years. Recovery left a larger number of employed individuals who were either uninsured or underinsured.

Between 1987 and 1989 there were significant changes in the character of the acute-care system. The most important were the stabilization and subsequent slight decrease in inpatient capacity and utilization and the rapid increase in services provided in the ambulatory and home care settings. Preferred provider organizations expanded at the expense of health maintenance organizations, and direct contracts for managed care between large industry and large health care providers were predicted for the future. Major reliance on the private sector for the provision of care and new initiatives was affirmed. State government continued the steady trend of greater involvement in health policy and health legislation.

Over the course of the study, a number of unexpected events occurred:

In a very short period of time, the profitability of selected hospitals improved remarkably. In 1987 there was widespread agreement that fundamental restrictions in both public and private third-party reimbursement practices would result in long-term financial stress and marginal profitability for most hospitals. The relatively short-lived recession simply added to the burden. The resurgence of seven of ten hospitals, as reflected in 1988 Medicare cost reports, seems remarkable.

At the end of the period, the traditional hospital and physician practice structures were beginning to dominate the alternative care systems. After six to ten years of steady development of health maintenance organizations and, subsequently, preferred provider organizations, they appeared poised to fight it out for the alternative market. Apparently hospitals, and perhaps group practices as well, have found ways of offering industry reduced cost care packages that threaten the alternative systems market.

The large multi-institutional systems held together by affiliation agreements and management contracts appear to be coming apart. Arguments made in the early 1980s about the mutual benefits of these arrangements to both the large supporting hospitals and the many smaller outlying ones seemed unassailable. Perhaps expectations on both sides have not been realized.

Hospitals are reported to be discontinuing home care services in favor of contracts with home care agencies. Hospital-based home care services seemed to answer needs for continuing care for patients discharged earlier than they would have been in a previous era and at the same time seemed to generate additional revenue. It appears that results have fallen short of this promise.

The nursing shortage that was of emergency proportions at the start of the study (1987) appeared to be slackening off in a remarkably brief period, the three years between 1987 and 1989. The size of the pool of available qualified nurses who simply refuse jobs they consider undesirable suggests that shortages might be quickly remedied by proffering more attractive conditions of employment. Those institutions that are able to offer these conditions appear to be solving this problem.

Conversely, several expected events failed to materialize during the study:

AIDS morbidity, although it escalated, did not progress at the rates originally projected. The slower than expected rise in AIDS morbidity may represent errors in original projections, the impact of preventive behavior, or combinations of these factors.

Despite the improvement in the economy and the reduction of unemployment in Harris County to under 6 percent, there was not a concomitant rise in the number of workers with health insurance, and those with insurance found themselves obligated to pay higher deductibles and copayments. That the work force would return to employment with fewer fringe benefits was totally unforeseen. Industry appears to be either unable or unwilling to continue to bear most of the costs of health care.

Physicians are readily available but not considered to be in surplus or to represent a significant problem by their numbers. Perhaps those observers who cited lower productivity in the work and life-styles of younger physicians were correct. A second factor may be the active marketing of a wide range of procedures performed by physicians in their offices rather than in hospitals.

The Role of Organized Groups and the Media

It is generally believed by local observers that business interests played an important role in many of these developments, but not a dominating one. The development of HMOs, PPOs, increased out-of-hospital care in the ambulatory or home setting, and, most recently, the direct managed-care arrangements between health care providers and corporations are all attributable to the combined pressure of both public and private insurers and business interests. Coalitions of voluntary agencies, foundations, and public health agencies are perceived as stronger advocates of public health concerns, such as improved outcomes of pregnancy among indigent populations.

Traditional provider groups, such as organized medicine and nursing and hospital representatives, continue to be influential. Third-party payers, business interests, and state government agencies are also important.

Universities are influential in those areas where academic health and medical care issues are decided.

In recent years, the dominant subject of media attention, as reflected in local newspapers, has been AIDS. Topics have ranged from features on AIDS as a medical and social problem, to difficulties plaguing Houston providers in presenting a coordinated front to funding sources, to limitations in availability of care. The plight of the homeless has been a recurrent subject in the media. Other subjects receiving major attention have included reductions in prenatal care and in clinic hours for patients with sexually transmitted diseases as a consequence of city health department budget cuts; small, inner-city hospital closures and attempts to finance their reopening; and the financial viability of the public hospital system.

The Future

Given the unexpected changes that occurred in the short period from 1987 to 1989, only modest predictions may be hazarded. The collective views of local observers suggest the continued dominance of insurer/hospital/corporate/group-practice interests and increases in managed-care contracts. In addition, the state legislature should be increasingly proactive as the health care cost problem affects individual voters, as the state's own expenses mount, and as providers and consumers alike demand state and federal responses.

State and local policymakers will continue to play a major role in indigent health care. However, the ultimate solution to problems of cost and of the uninsured will probably still be viewed as a federal task.

Interview Panel

Madeleine Appel, council coordinator for City Council member Eleanor Tinsley
Howard C. Allen, chief, Bureau of Long Term Care, Texas Department of Health
Spencer Bayles, M.D., psychiatrist; member of the Mental Health Needs Council (representing the Harris County Medical Society); former medical director, HCA Belle Park Hospital
Becky Beechinor, program administrator, Licensing Section, Texas Department of Health
Lan Bentsen, businessman; chairman, Texas Coalition for Maternal and Child Health; national trustee, March of Dimes
Honorable Chet Brooks, senator, Texas State Senate
Madgelean Bush, director, Martin Luther King, Jr., Community Center; former board member, Riverside General Hospital
Richard Butler, chief, Bureau of Long Term Care, Texas Department of Health
D. Claghorn, M.D., psychiatrist; director, Clinical Research Associates

Richard Durbin, former chief executive officer, Harris County Hospital District
Mamie Ewing, regional administrator, Texas Department of Human Services
Stanton Fischer, M.D., physician-in-chief, Kelsey-Seybold Clinic
Garrett Graham, president and chief executive officer, Greater Houston Hospital
    Council
Carroll Gregory, program administrator, Health Maintenance Organization Pro-
    gram, Texas Department of Health
Tom Hyslop, M.D., director, Harris County Health Department
Edith Irby Jones, M.D., internist, private practice
Joanne Kennedy, director of insurance related activities, Texas State Board of Insur-
    · ance
Claudia Langguth, former regional administrator, Texas Department of Human
    Services
Shelly Liss, M.D., medical director, Department of Physical and Rehabilitative
    Medicine, Memorial Southwest Hospital
Rachel Lucas, executive director, Chicano Family Center; former chair, Harris
    County Hospital District Council of Consumers
Larry Mathis, chief executive officer, Methodist Hospital
Lois Moore, president and chief executive officer, Harris County Hospital District
S. Kelley Moseley, Dr.P.H., president, S.K.M. Associates
Sandra S. Person, executive director, Houston Area Health Care Coalition
John Ribble, M.D., former acting president, The University of Texas Health Science
    Center at Houston; dean, The University of Texas Medical School at Houston
Robert F. Schaper, president and chief executive officer, Tomball Regional Hospital
Patricia Starck, D.S.N., dean, The University of Texas School of Nursing at Houston
John R. Strawn, M.D., internist, partner and member of the Executive Committee,
    Medical Clinic of Houston
Kay Swint, director, Managed Care, West Oaks Hospital System
Marty Tullis, administrator, Harris County Psychiatric Center
Richard Wainerdi, Ph.D., president, Texas Medical Center
Craig Watson, president, Visiting Nurses Association
Robert Weinberger, Ph.D., clinical psychologist; president, Weinberger, Hall and
    Associates, P.C.
Ken Wine, vice president, Memorial Care System

Bibliography

A Commonwealth Fund Paper: What to Do About the Nursing Shortage (New York: The
    Commonwealth Fund, 1989).
American Hospital Association Guide to the Health Care Field (Chicago: American Hos-
    pital Association, 1977–1989).
County and City Data Book (Washington, D.C.: U.S. Department of Commerce, Bu-
    reau of the Census, 1988).
Family Health Services Statistics, Mimeograph (Houston: Department of Health
    and Human Services, 1988).

Fiscal Year 1990 Budget (Houston: Department of Health and Human Services, 1990).

Geographic Profile of Employment and Unemployment (Washington, D.C.: U.S. Department of Labor, 1987).

The Health of Houston (Houston: Department of Health and Human Services, 1980–84, 1981–85).

Hospital Cost Reports, Unpublished Data (Washington, D. C.: U.S. Department of Health and Human Services, Health Care Finance Administration, 1988).

Hospital Ownership and Bed Study (Houston: Greater Houston Hospital Council, 1986–1989).

Hospital Statistics (Chicago: American Hospital Association, 1977–1989).

Houston Chronicle, selected articles, July 1988 through December 15, 1989.

Houston Facts (Houston: Greater Houston Partnership, 1990).

Houston Metropolitan Area Employment Statistics and Outlook for Job Creation (Austin: Texas Employment Commission, Economic Research and Analysis Department, 1989).

Houston Post, selected articles, July 1988 through December 15, 1989.

Patient Services Summary, Mimeograph (Houston: Harris County Hospital District, 1988).

Personal Health Services Statistics, Mimeograph (Houston: Harris County Health Department, 1988).

Physician Characteristics and Distribution in the U.S. (Chicago: American Medical Association, 1978–1989).

Population Changes by Ethnicity: 1980 vs. 1990, Mimeograph (Houston: Department of Health and Human Services, Bureau of Health Planning, 1991).

Population Data System, State Health Planning and Resource Development (Austin: Texas Department of Health, Bureau of State Health Data and Policy Analysis, 1986).

Special Texas Census (Austin: Texas Department of Human Services, 1985).

State and Metropolitan Area Data Book (Washington, D.C.: U.S. Department of Commerce, Bureau of the Census, 1986).

Supply of Physicians, Dentists and Registered Nurses in Harris County, Mimeograph (Houston: Center for Health Policy Studies, The University of Texas School of Public Health, 1988).

Texas Almanac and State Industrial Guide (Dallas: A.H. Belo Corporation, 1989).

Texas Vital Statistics (Austin: Texas Department of Health, 1987).

Texas HMO Status Report, Mimeograph (Austin: Texas State Board of Insurance, 1988).

The Houston Sourcebook (Houston: Greater Houston Partnership, 1991).

Vital Statistics of the United States (Hyattsville, MD: U.S. Department of Health and Human Services, 1988).

6

Parallels, Differences,
and Prospects

Eli Ginzberg

This concluding chapter highlights some of the principal themes that emerged from the study of systemic change in each of the four metropolitan areas during the 1980s. To provide a framework for the parallels and differences that were discerned, as well as the prospects for reform in the years ahead, the findings are subsumed under four headings: the changing demand for health care services; health care delivery—hospitals, clinics, physicians; alternative delivery systems, and the changing resource base and public policy.

The Changing Demand for Health Care Services

All of the cities that were studied underwent considerable changes in their population profiles and economic bases, which altered materially the demand for health care services in their respective metropolitan areas. Los Angeles experienced the most rapid increase in population, which was heavily concentrated in the lower income groups. The overall result was an increased proportion of poor and near-poor residents relative to the more affluent. Houston's population declined somewhat with the onset of the oil recession early in the decade, only to expand once the economy rebounded after 1987. There, too, the proportion of low-income minority groups, particularly Hispanics, increased substantially. In absolute terms, the resident populations of Chicago and New York remained more or less constant; however, these metros experienced similar increases in the proportion of low-income families.

In sum, at the decade's end the four metros faced the challenge of meeting the demand for health care services from growing numbers of persons who were not insured, had shallow insurance, or were enrolled in Medicaid. The poor and near poor were heavily dependent on public hospitals and clinics and on charity care provided by nonprofit hospitals. Much of what transpired in the 1980s was linked to the ability and willingness of these providers to respond to the growing needs of the indigent and the uninsured.

Closely related factors that contributed to the expansion of demand were the proliferation of new morbidities, particularly HIV infection and crack addiction; the exacerbation of social pathologies, such as homelessness and untreated mental illness; and the influx of illegal immigrants. New York and Los Angeles both had disproportionately large numbers of AIDS patients and were magnets for illegal immigrants. The largest recipient of immigrants was Los Angeles; New York followed with about 100,000 entrants annually.

The ability of the four metros to meet the expanded health care demands of low income groups was influenced by the vicissitudes of their respective economies. Houston, as has been noted, underwent a serious recession for most of the 1980s. Chicago's economic base was weakened early in the decade by the steep decline in its manufacturing sector and the continuing out-migration to the suburbs of its more affluent residents. The 1980s were, in general, favorable for New York until the end of the decade, when the consequences of the stock market crash of October 1987 became increasingly visible in losses of both jobs and income. Although Los Angeles enjoyed a generally salubrious economic climate throughout the 1980s, some of its high-wage manufacturing was replaced by low-wage industries.

Overall, Chicago and Houston were more seriously threatened by the state of their economies in meeting the health care demands of burgeoning low income populations than were New York and Los Angeles. The latter, however, were confronted with steeper increases in demand that were generated in New York by rampant medical and social pathologies and in Los Angeles by large inflows of impoverished immigrants.

Health Care Delivery—Hospitals, Clinics, Physicians

We have noted that powerful common trends contributed to the increased demand for health care services by the poor and uninsured in all four regions. However, when it comes to the structure and responsiveness of their respective delivery systems, considerable variation is found. A significant differentiator was the scale and scope of the public sector. For generations, New York has operated a large, comprehensive network of municipal hospitals, clinics, chronic-care institutions, and ambulatory facilities. Los Angeles has a less well-elaborated public system, and Houston and Chicago, especially the latter, lag very far behind.

Another important differentiator was the status of the non-profit sector. Numerous nonprofit community hospitals that had long served the inner-city residents of Chicago were forced to close, and parallel closures (though to a lesser extent) occurred in Los Angeles County. Houston lost just two small acute-care hospitals. In New York, there was little left to lose following an aggressive state policy in the 1970s that reduced the city's bed capacity by approximately 30 percent. The number of hospitals in Chicago and Los Angeles that ceased operating during the 1980s would have been even larger had not some benefitted from their membership in a hospital network or system that occasionally applied earnings from profitable suburban facilities to maintain weak inner-city institutions.

It is worth noting that Houston is the only area studied in which the hospital sector is not dominated by nonprofit institutions. As far back as the 1970s, for-profit hospitals have led in number and bed capacity. However, the most prestigious health care complex, the Texas Medical Center, consists exclusively of nonprofit institutions—the two AHCs, the University of Texas and Baylor, and most of their affiliated hospitals.

Transformations on the hospital front affected not only the provision of care to the poor but services for the insured population as well. In Chicago, many of the leading institutions in the inner city, such as the teaching hospitals of Northwestern University and Rush, forged alliances with suburban hospitals to enlarge their referral bases and to realize other mutual benefits. The same was true for several of the larger, church-sponsored networks that had been founded in the inner city.

Houston again was somewhat different. Several of its leading health institutions had developed linkages with hospitals elsewhere in Texas and in other southern states. By the mid- to late 1980s, however, many of these had been terminated, in large part because the nuclear institutions were unduly exposed to malpractice suits.

In the course of the 1980s, New York hospitals that had previously attracted a significant proportion of their admissions by referral from the suburbs and beyond found this flow reduced by as much as one-third as a result of the expansion and increasing sophistication of the outlying hospitals. The preference of suburban physicians to admit patients to local hospitals was reinforced by the fear on the part of many suburban residents of exposure to the deteriorating conditions in the city, in particular, crime.

Hospital occupancy in New York—as throughout the nation—declined substantially during the decade due to numerous interacting factors including prospective reimbursement, the shift to ambulatory surgery, the shortened average length of stay, and other developments. In the late

1980s, however, hospital admissions unexpectedly spiked and (like city traffic) became virtually gridlocked, with many institutions operating at over 90 percent of capacity. The severe overcrowding was attributed to continuing pressure by the state department of health to force the hospitals to reduce their bed complements; to increased demand generated by AIDS, substance abuse, homelessness, and the deinstitutionalization of the mentally ill; and, for a time, to an acute shortage of nurses. Although occupancy rates in most of the nonprofit and for-profit hospitals in Chicago, Los Angeles, and Houston, in conformity with the country at large, ranged from 50 to 60 percent (somewhat higher in major teaching institutions), their public hospitals operated close to capacity and, in the case of Los Angeles, often well above.

With respect to total bed complements, only Houston saw an expansion in the public sector, which was a result of the rebuilding of two of its three hospitals with a net addition of 300 beds. Yet despite the new construction and the enlarged capacity, the public hospitals in Houston were not able to do much more, in meeting the health needs of the poor, than care for a large number of obstetrics patients and trauma cases. Many more of the poor who needed and might have profited from hospital treatment could not be accommodated. In stark contrast, the steadily deteriorating Cook County Hospital in Chicago remained the only public hospital available to all of the poor residing in the city.

All four metros supported a number of clinics, hospital-based and free standing, which provided a considerable volume of ambulatory care to the poor. In both Los Angeles and Houston, all patients, except for the poorest, were expected to pay on a sliding scale, depending on their income, for the services that they received. The public hospital system in New York, unlike that in Los Angeles and Houston, did not make any serious efforts to extract payment from the uninsured population that sought care at its facilities.

As the decade advanced, many hospitals that had initially participated in trauma networks, particularly in Chicago and Los Angeles, withdrew from those networks because of the potential financial losses entailed in admitting and treating seriously injured individuals, many with little or no insurance coverage. In Houston, by the end of the decade, only one hospital, a public institution, routinely accepted serious cases brought in by the emergency medical services (EMS). Similarly, a growing number of nonprofit hospitals in each of the metros sought ways to limit or close their emergency rooms because of the substantial number of admissions through this conduit for whom there was no source of reimbursement.

In low income neighborhoods in all four areas, the poor and the near-poor obtained much of their ambulatory care from local practitioners, many of them foreign medical graduates. Most of these physicians developed active practices treating large numbers of patients, but the quality of care that they provided was often marginal. In general, they were not affiliated with the local hospital(s) and did not follow the care of their patients once they were hospitalized.

The prevailing perception in the four metros was that each had a sufficient number of practitioners and specialists, and there was some evidence of selected surpluses. But without exception, the proportion of physicians to population ranged widely, from 1:150-250 in affluent sections to 1:17, 500 in poverty areas.

Alternative Delivery Systems

Throughout the 1980s, there was widespread activity focused on the elaboration of innovative delivery systems to replace fee-for-service practice. Concrete developments, however, varied greatly among the four metros.

In Los Angeles, the birthplace of the modern HMO with the establishment of the Ross-Loos Clinic in 1929, HMOs continued their rapid growth and were joined in the early 1980s by PPOs, which proliferated rapidly. As a result, the health care market became highly competitive in the course of a few years. The intensity of the competition in Los Angeles was fueled by the continuing decline in hospital occupancy rates. Under mounting pressure to attract patients, hospitals were willing to offer special discounts to secure additional admissions. Further, because physicians were the key to admissions and also played a major role in generating ambulatory care income, hospitals made concerted efforts to recruit and retain attending staff who could contribute to their patient flows. As the decade progressed, the hospitals also experimented with a variety of joint activities with physician groups as a means of increasing their work loads and revenues. Some of these arrangements were clearly at the fringe of propriety and legitimacy.

Because for-profit hospitals and HMOs had realized their greatest expansion in the Los Angeles and Houston areas, it is important to note that the introduction of the DRGs (in 1983), which coincided with a fall off in hospital admissions, resulted in serious financial difficulties for a number of for-profit chains. This situation was especially the case for several for-profit HMO chains whose entrepreneurial optimism had led to unsound expansion. Maxicare was an outstanding example.

In Chicago the situation was different. Although HMOs had only a peripheral presence at the start of the decade, in the succeeding few years—for reasons that are not altogether clear—the HMO sector spurted. Enrollments rose to about 25 percent and in some areas were even higher. During the second half of the decade, however, HMO growth not only leveled off but actually declined as many enrollees and physicians became disenchanted with the services and operations of the HMOs. Some of the new delivery systems found that they had expanded too rapidly, that they were deficient in administrative and managerial skills, and that they were faced with financial difficulties necessitating contraction and consolidation.

New York provides a quite different scenario: In that city there were strenuous efforts to establish innovative delivery systems but little short- or long-run success. In 1986, the state legislature rescinded its ban on for-profit HMOs and thus cleared the way for action by several national chains that targeted New York as a promising site for enrollment growth. Sizable sums were invested in the attempt to penetrate the metropolitan market, but except for some moderate successes in the nearby suburbs, the city proper proved almost totally inhospitable. Eventually there was no option but to withdraw.

Failure of the for-profit HMOs to establish a profitable niche in the New York market was certainly overdetermined. However, some of the likely causative factors can be identified: the overall satisfaction of the insured population with its broad choice among the city's vast supply of experienced physicians in every specialty; the indifferent reputation of the Health Insurance Plan (HIP), the city's oldest HMO (nonprofit), which had been in operation since the 1940s; and the difficulties and high cost of finding optimal or even suitable locations for a prospective HMO clientele.

In Houston, the HMO movement made some modest gains by the early 1980s, but even at its peak it never matched the experience either of Los Angeles or Chicago. Its indolent growth may be attributed to the defensive tactics that the city's conservative physician community adopted in order to retain its hegemony. Physicians in Houston offered employers new cost-saving arrangements for the provision of ambulatory care to large numbers of patients, which inhibited HMO growth, ironically at the employers' expense. Further, many of the hospitals in the Houston area were willing to provide the employer community with new contractual arrangements, and a corresponding savings was realized from the quicker put-through of inpatients and the shift to more outpatient treatment.

Brief reference needs to be made to PPOs, which originated and enjoyed their most sustained expansion in southern California but had counterparts in the other three metros as well. Even now (in mid-1991), it is difficult to assess the scale, scope, and success of the PPOs. At a minimum, it seems safe to conclude that by offering consumers greater choice at the point of service, admittedly for an additional cost, they have interrupted the earlier growth of HMOs. Further, they appear to be serving as one of the building blocks for the resurgence of insurance companies that offer employers joint-risk contracts with lower premium costs in exchange for the utilization of efficient physicians and hospitals. The growth potential of this latest innovation on the delivery front is as yet uncertain.

One of the disappointments of the 1980s was the desultory progress of HMOs in enrolling Medicare and Medicaid patients, despite the inducement of liberalized reimbursement for Medicare beneficiaries by the federal government. Even in southern California where Kaiser has had long and successful experience in operating HMOs, the number of federally entitled patients that the plan accepts is severely restricted.

The state of New York has made a few attempts to enroll Medicaid patients in HMOs, but the resistance, especially in New York City, from the Medicaid population and the physicians who treat them has been formidable. These efforts were reintensified in 1991 with the hope of saving money and improving the quality of care that the Medicaid population receives.

The Changing Resource Base

The overarching financial reality of the 1980s was the steady acceleration in total spending for health care, which rose nationally from around $250 billion at the start of the decade (1980) to $604 billion at its end (1989), notwithstanding the precipitous deceleration in the general inflation rate after 1982. Although each of the principal payers—the federal government, state governments, and employers—initiated a large number of efforts to control their expenditures, the end results indicate that they did not succeed. Without their efforts, however, the total dollars spent on health care would unquestionably have been greater.

The combination of reduced hospital admissions, shorter lengths of stay, pressures to offer special discounts (particularly in California), the shift to a prospective payment system by Medicare, the introduction of competitive contracting for Medicaid in both California and Illinois, and the growth of the uninsured and underinsured populations everywhere placed the nongovernmental hospital system in each metropolitan area under increasing financial stress. The inner-city hospitals, in particular, were faced with the need to admit disproportionate numbers of Medicaid recipients and uninsured patients. Because the prospective reimbursement scale that the federal government initially adopted for Medicare was favorable to hospitals, it was a few years before hospital patient care margins were seriously reduced. By 1990, however, a growing number and proportion of hospitals, particularly in New York and Chicago, were operating with negative margins.

The financial pressures confronting many nonprofit acute-care hospitals have been exacerbated by the practice in all four states of skimping on

Medicaid reimbursements by both narrowing the scope of coverage and delaying payment. To make matters worse, when the public hospitals were unable to respond effectively to the emergent needs of the poor and the uninsured, many nonprofit hospitals located in the inner cities made efforts to fill the breach, and some were brought to the brink of, or actually forced into, bankruptcy as a result.

Compounding the foregoing has been the inadequate financial support, particularly in Chicago and Los Angeles, for public sector hospitals and clinics. The situation in Houston is not much better because of the very low proportion of the poverty population (just over one-third) that is eligible for Medicaid. New York is the only state that can claim to have been reasonably responsive in funding its public sector health facilities. However, the city has been confronted by the extraordinary demand for new types of care that not only are costly but also have compromised its ability to provide the services traditionally needed by the poor.

Rising financial pressures on the chief component of the health care system—the acute-care hospital—are also partly responsible for the failure of the nonhospital sector—nursing homes, home care, hospices—to enjoy significant expansion or improvement in quality during the 1980s. Of these three types of service, home care, which is funded principally by households (except in New York City, where Medicaid expends $1 billion annually on its home care program) fared the best in terms of growth and the sophistication of services available at home to the chronically ill.

The final questions that need to be addressed are whether and how the increasingly stressed and strained financial environment was reflected in new public policy and programmatic initiatives. The simple answer is that health issues and health policy failed to elicit serious or sustained attention among the media, the public, the politicians, or the state legislatures. This is not to say that the media did not periodically address the AIDS pandemic or the threats and dangers from the growing use of cocaine and crack. However, health policy resolutions to systemic issues, such as proposals for extending insurance coverage to the entire population and effective cost controls, failed to engage the public sufficiently to effect legislative action.

In none of the four states—New York, Illinois, Texas, or California—did either the governor or the state legislature take the bold step of instituting a large-scale reform of the state's health care system. In the whole of the United States, only the state of Massachusetts undertook such an effort, and it soon foundered in the wake of the economic recession that engulfed the state almost immediately thereafter. Inasmuch as the states are responsible for the smallest share of the funds that flow into health care—10 to 13 percent as opposed to 25 to 32 percent contributed by the federal government, employers, and households—it is questionable that even a large and affluent state would have been in a position to remodel its health care system in any fundamental respect.

Such remodeling is contingent upon a broad political consensus among the federal government, state government, employers, and the public, and it is this consensus that has yet to develop. In the interim, the federal government, besieged by growing budgetary deficits, has decided to leave health policy innovation to the private sector and the states. Neither of these entities has found the key to forging an effective alliance with the federal government, which alone can speed remedial action. The early 1990s suggest that more time must pass before the preconditions are established for a collective alignment of all the interested parties to take action that will assure both universal coverage and cost containment. How much additional time is needed before the nation will grapple with these imperatives? That question remains open.

Contributors

Howard S. Berliner, Sc.D., is Associate Professor and Chair of the Department of Health Services Management and Policy, Graduate School of Management and Urban Policy, The New School for Social Research, New York.

E. Richard Brown, Ph.D., is Professor of Public Health at the University of California, Los Angeles.

Geraldine Dallek, M.P.H., is Executive Director of the Medicare Advocacy Project, Inc. in Los Angeles, California.

Eli Ginzberg, Ph.D., is Director of The Eisenhower Center for the Conservation of Human Resources, Columbia University.

Virginia C. Kennedy, Ph.D., is Associate Professor of Management and Policy Sciences, School of Public Health, The University of Texas Health Science Center at Houston.

Hardy D. Loe, Jr., M.D., M.P.H., is Associate Professor of Community Health, School of Public Health, The University of Texas Health Science Center at Houston.

Frank I. Moore, Ph.D., is Associate Professor of Management and Policy Sciences, School of Public Health, The University of Texas Health Science Center at Houston.

Miriam Ostow, M.A., is Senior Research Scholar at The Eisenhower Center for the Conservation of Human Resources, Columbia University.

J. Warren Salmon, Ph.D., is Professor and Department Head, Pharmacy Administration, and Professor of Health Resources and Management, School of Public Health, The University of Illinois at Chicago.

About the Book

The decade of the 1980s promised basic reform in the provision of health care services. Ronald Reagan, newly elected to the presidency on a pledge to minimize the role of government in domestic affairs, committed his administration to the pursuit of free-market strategies as the panacea for the costliness and inefficiency besetting the nation's health care system. Official and private rhetoric was replete with proposals for systemic change fueled by the competitive forces that would be unleashed by deregulation.

Once the federal government yielded its long-held place as innovator and reformer, it was inevitable that the states would be catapulted into positions of greater prominence in the shaping of health care policy. This book assesses the changes that have actually occurred in the U.S. health care system, analyzing the nation's four largest metropolitan centers, which together with their states account for 74 million persons, or roughly one-third of the nation's population.

The study delineates specific developments within each metro area, attempting to capture and analyze the many differences and the many parallels among the four that might illuminate the dynamics and the contours of change in the health care system. Among the areas selected for investigation are the following:

- Alternative responses to the growing surplus of acute-care hospital beds
- The potentiators of, and the impediments to, the elaboration of HMOs and other innovative forms of health care delivery
- Public and private responses to the uncompensated care issue
- The establishment of new ambulatory care facilities and their interaction with existing hospitals
- The responses of both the governmental and nongovernmental sectors to the growing surplus of physicians and the supply of other medical personnel
- The impact of pressures imposed by declining hospital admissions and early discharges on the nursing home and home health care sectors
- The principal consequences for local academic health centers (AHCs) of the more price-competitive environment and the shift from inpatient to ambulatory treatment
- The degree of satisfaction/disappointment among the local business coalitions with progress toward their major goals and the modification of these goals with experience
- Identification of health care issues that commanded the attention of the press, the public, and political groups, and the action taken in response to them

Changing U.S. Health Care represents a major attempt to contrast the rhetoric and predictions of the 1980s with the realities facing the health care system today.

206

Index

March of Dimes Birth Defects Foundation, 163, 188
Martin Luther King Hospital (L.A.), 115, 117–118
Maryville Academy (Chicago), 60
Massachusetts, 203
Maternal and child health, 181, 182, 187
Maternal and Infant Health Improvement Act (Tex.), 189
Maternity care, 117, 172, 187
Maxicare (HMO), 28, 29, 68, 109, 110
MCHC. *See* Metropolitan Chicago Healthcare Council
M. D. Anderson Hospital and Tumor Institute, 162
Measles, 37, 84, 124–125, 182
Media. *See under* Health care services
Medicaid, 3, 6, 10, 22, 30, 159, 176, 196–197
  and ambulatory care, 64
  eligibility, 34, 89, 187
  expenditures, 7, 76
  and immigrants, 106
  payment reduction, 2, 7, 43, 63, 75
  payments, 79, 80, 181, 186
  physician reimbursement, 50
  and pregnant women and children, 2, 43, 106
  and states, 2, 7, 8, 30, 42, 52, 76, 187, 188, 202–203
  See also under Chicago; Houston; Los Angeles; New York City
Medi-Cal, 103, 106, 110, 111, 112–113, 114, 115, 118–119, 123, 127, 128, 130–131, 133, 134, 139, 142, 143, 144, 145, 146, 150
Medical Assistance, No Grant (MANG), 86
Medical infrastructure, 13, 18–19, 23, 116
Medically indigent adults (MIAs), 112, 113, 119
Medically Indigent Services Program (MISP), 113
Medical societies, 4, 50–52
Medical technology, 3, 18, 20, 21, 24, 31, 63, 65, 103, 116, 145, 173
Medicare, 3, 6, 68, 159
  amendments (1988), 75
  B, 4
  and catastrophic illness, 10, 142
  costs, 4, 7
  fee and volume controls, 4
  and home health care, 144–145
  and hospice care, 146
  payments, 66, 79, 80, 85, 143, 173, 186

See also under Chicago; Houston; Los Angeles; New York City
Melnick, G. A., 103
Memorial Hospital System (Houston), 167
Memorial Southwest Hospital (Houston), 167
Mental illness, 16, 21, 24, 37, 55, 77, 118, 120, 162, 171, 197, 199
Methodist Hospital (Houston), 167, 168
Methodist Hospital (L.A.), 139
MetLife (HMO), 29(table), 68
Metro (HMO), 29(table)
Metropolitan Chicago Healthcare Council (MCHC), 43, 50, 70, 74, 85, 86
Metropolitan Planning Council (Chicago), 54
MIAs. *See* Medically indigent adults
Microsurgery, 25
Midwest Business Group on Health, 51
Miles Square Health Center (Chicago), 88, 89
MISP. *See* Medically Indigent Services Program
Montefiore Medical Center (N.Y.C.), 18, 28
Mount Sinai Medical Center (N.Y.C.), 18, 22, 23, 28, 34
Mt. Sinai-North Hospital (Chicago), 59, 64, 86
MRI. *See* Magnetic resonance imaging

National Aeronautics and Space Center (Tex.), 161
National health insurance, 151
National Health Planning and Resources Development Act (1974), 188
National health policy, 190
National Medical Care Expenditures Survey (1977), 85
National Medical Enterprises (NME), 6, 48, 126, 133, 138
National Medical Enterprises/University of Southern California (NME/USC) Medical School hospital, 137, 138–139
National Physicians Housestaff Association, 52
NCB. *See* North Central Bronx Hospital
Near Westside Medical Center (Chicago), 60
Neonatal intensive care, 81, 84, 172
New Jersey, 23, 35
New Provident Community Organization (Chicago), 61

.